Nutrition for
Veterinary Technicians
and Nurses

Nutrition for
Veterinary Technicians and Nurses

Ann Wortinger, LVT, VTS (ECC)

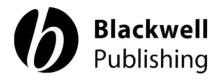

Blackwell
Publishing

Ann Wortinger, LVT, VTS (ECC), is the program coordinator for the Veterinary Technology Program at Wayne State University, teaching clinical pathology. With 16 years experience in Internal medicine, Ann founded and coordinated care for the nutritional support service at a major specialty/referral hospital. She obtained her specialty certification in emergency and critical care in 2000, and is a founding member of the Academy of Internal Medicine of Veterinary Technicians, experienced in general practice, emergency and specialty medicine.

Blackwell Publishing Professional
2121 State Avenue, Ames, Iowa 50014, USA

Orders: 1-800-862-6657
Office: 1-515-292-0140
Fax: 1-515-292-3348
Web site: www.blackwellprofessional.com

Blackwell Publishing Ltd
9600 Garsington Road, Oxford OX4 2DQ, UK
Tel.: +44 (0)1865 776868

Blackwell Publishing Asia
550 Swanston Street, Carlton, Victoria 3053, Australia
Tel.: +61 (0)3 8359 1011

First edition, 2007

Library of Congress Cataloging-in-Publication Data

Wortinger, Ann.
   Nutrition for veterinary technicians / Ann Wortinger. — 1st ed.
      p. ; cm.
Includes bibliographical references.
ISBN-13: 978-0-8138-2913-5 (alk. paper)
ISBN-10: 0-8138-2913-5 (alk. paper)
1. Dogs—Food. 2. Cats—Food. 3. Animal nutrition.
      I. Title.
   [DNLM: 1. Animal Nutrition. 2. Cats. 3. Dogs. SF 95 W932n
2007]
   SF427.4.W67 2007
   636.089'32—dc22
                                        2006025800

The last digit is the print number: 9 8 7 6 5 4 3 2 1

TABLE OF CONTENTS

SECTION 3   Feeding Management for Dogs and Cats   129

Nutrition is an area of veterinary medicine in which it is very easy for the technician to have an active role. Many of the commercial food producers have concentrated on educating technicians on nutrition. There are nutrition tracks at most national conferences, as well as online learning programs.

As with any other area of education, you still need to know the basics to understand what is being taught, and unfortunately, this is often not addressed for technicians. While chemistry, microbiology, and math are required at most schools, even these do not adequately address basic animal nutrition. We all are taught the basic nutrients in a diet—water, protein, fats, and carbohydrates—but we need to know how they work together, what happens to them inside the body, and what changes occur with aging.

So where does this leave a technician who wants to know more about nutrition, who wants to really understand what is going on inside the animal? Usually, they start by going through the available veterinary nutrition books, but the first chapter can be overwhelming. These books often provide more details than a technician needs or wants to know; one tends to get lost in these details and miss the basic points. Human nutrition books do not address the unique nutritional needs of either dogs or cats, although they can often address basic nutrition in a less technical manner. Some people enroll in an online program, but the basics are often missing from these and referencing these later can be difficult. I love having reference books available whenever I have a question or need clarification on a point of interest, and I often have questions and need clarification!

I have plowed through nutrition books from the very basic pet owner books to the extremely technical veterinary books; all of them have something to offer, but will everyone read long enough to understand it? I was very fortunate to have a number of veterinarians who were willing to explain the points I did not understand, to correct me when I misunderstood a concept, and to direct me to areas that I may find interesting. Without them, I would have had a much more difficult time understanding and utilizing nutrition in our day-to-day practice. After all, that is the ultimate goal of nutrition, isn't it?

My goal in writing this book was to provide a resource for technicians that was both relevant and technical, but also understandable and usable. This is not a dummied-down version of a veterinary nutrition book, but one that focuses on the unique interests of technicians and how we use nutrition in practice and at home.

This book is organized into three sections. Section 1 addresses the basics of nutrition by looking at energy and nutrients; how the individual nutrients of water, carbohydrates, fats, proteins, vitamins, and minerals are utilized by the body; digestions and absorption of these nutrients; and, finally, energy balance. Section 2 covers nutritional requirements for cats and dogs by going through the history and regulation of pet foods, understanding how to read pet food labels, understanding nutrient content and types of foods and how they differ, and evaluating raw food diets, preservatives, and homemade diets. Finally, section 3 covers different feeding regimens and body condition scoring (both definition and use) and takes feeding from pregnancy and lactation through neonatal, growth, and adult maintenance feeding and into geriatrics. Section 3 also covers feeding for performance animals, special feeding requirement for cats, nutrition myths, the use of nutritional support, and assisted feeding techniques. Each section builds on the information covered in previous sections, allowing for practical use of the information learned.

My cats are not thrilled when I start calculating caloric intake, nutrient distribution, or metabolizable energy. But they will ultimately benefit from my knowledge, as have innumerable clients, patients, coworkers, and students.

My hope is that with this book you will come to appreciate the important role nutrition plays in veterinary medicine, through both prevention and therapeutic use. You will have a better understanding of basic digestion, nutrient use by the body, and how food can affect our patients from the prenatal period through their death (hopefully, many years down the line). And you will bring nutrition into your practice and use it to improve the quality of care that is provided to your patients. Nutrition is an ever-evolving field in veterinary medicine, and I hope this book serves as a stepping stone for future learning. I love veterinary nutrition, and I hope that you will come to love it, too!

ACKNOWLEDGEMENTS

With any writing project, there are those who suffer during the creative process. My husband, Todd, has suffered the most since he lost half of his office so I could have a place to work. He also had to listen to my exciting conversation when I would finally surface after writing all day. Who really wants to hear about vitamins and lipids over dinner? My thanks go to him for all his support and for lending an ear when he really didn't want to know what I was talking about to begin with.

My thanks also go to Dr. Ned Kuehn for sparking my interest in nutrition and allowing me the leeway to pursue it in clinical practice. Although he did not want to hear about vitamins and lipids either, he was always there to answer my unending questions and allowed me to use what I learned to improve the outcome for our patients.

To Kathe Koja, the best kind of client. As a writer, your editorial help was invaluable, your support welcome, and your enthusiasm appreciated.

To my feline editorial staff; Cheyenne-Abyssinian extraordinaire, Daisy, Lily, and Rose—the Flower Children. You ladies had the unfailing ability to know exactly which text I was currently working out of, or would need next. You very kindly marked it with your furry bodies. How does anyone work without a feline editorial staff?

1

Basics of Nutrition

1

Nutrients and Energy

Animals, unlike plants, are unable to generate their own energy, and they require a balanced diet to grow normally, maintain health once they are mature, reproduce, and perform physical work (Case et al., 2000). Plants are able to convert solar energy into carbohydrates thorough a process called photosynthesis, but they also require water, vitamins, and minerals for optimal growth and production. To obtain their energy, animals either eat plants or eat other animals that eat plants (Case et al., 2000).

Nutrients

For animals, energy is provided in the diet through nutrients. Nutrients are components of the diet that have specific functions within the body and contribute to growth, tissue maintenance, and optimal health (Case et al., 2000). Essential nutrients are those components that cannot be synthesized by the body at a rate adequate to meet the body's needs, so they must be included in the diet. These nutrients are used as structural components for bone and muscle, enhance or are involved in metabolism, transport substances such as oxygen and electrolytes, maintain normal body temperature, and supply energy (Case et al., 2000; Gross et al., 2000). Nonessential nutrients can be synthesized by the body and can be obtained either through production by the body or through the diet (Case et al., 2000). Nutrients are further divided into six major categories: water, carbohydrates, proteins, fats, vitamins, and minerals.

Energy is not one of the major nutrients, but after water it is the most critical component of the diet, with energy needs always being the first requirement to be met in an animal's diet (Case et al., 2000). After energy needs have been met, nutrients become available for other metabolic functions (Case et al., 2000). Approximately 50% to 80% of the dry matter of a dog's or cat's diet is used for energy (Case et al., 2000). The body obtains energy from nutrients through oxidation of the chemical bonds found in proteins, carbohydrates, and fats (Gross et al., 2000). This oxidation occurs during digestion, absorption, and transport into the body's cells (Gross et al., 2000). The most important energy-containing compound that is produced is adenosine triphosphate (ATP) (Gross et al., 2000).

The biochemical reactions that occur within the body either use or release energy. Anabolic reactions require energy for completion, and catabolic reactions release energy upon completion (Gross et al., 2000). ATP and other energy-trapping compounds pick up part of the energy release from one process and transfer it to the other processes (Gross et al., 2000). This energy is used for pumping ions, for molecular synthesis, and to activate contractile proteins—these three processes essentially describe the total use of energy by the animal (Gross et al., 2000). Without the energy supplied through the diet, these reactions would not occur and death would follow (Gross et al., 2000).

ATP is the usable form of energy for the body, but it is not a good form of energy storage because it is used quickly after being produced (Gross et al., 2000). Glycogen and triglycerides are better storage forms of energy (Gross et al., 2000). In fasting animals, when the body needs energy, it uses glycogen first, stored fat second, and amino acids from body protein as a last resort (Gross et al., 2000).

Gross Energy

The total amount of potential energy contained within a diet is called gross energy (GE). GE in food is determined by burning the food in a bomb calorimeter and measuring the total amount of heat produced. Unfortunately, animals are not able to use 100% of the energy contained in a food; some of it is lost during digestion and assimilation of nutrients, as well as in urine, feces, respiration, and production of heat (Case et al., 2000; Gross et al., 2000).

Digestible Energy

Digestible energy (DE) refers to the energy available for absorption across the intestinal mucosa; the energy lost is found in the feces. Metabolizable energy (ME) is the amount of energy actually available to the tissue for use; the energy lost is found in the feces and urine. ME is the value most often used to express the energy content in pet foods (Case et al., 2000; Gross et al., 2000).

When GE values are readjusted for digestibility and urinary losses, ME values of 3.5 kcal/g are assigned to proteins and carbohydrates and of 8.5 kcal/g are assigned to fats; these values are called modified Atwater factors (Case et al., 2000; Gross et al., 2000).

The ME of a diet or food ingredient depends on both the nutrient composition of the food and the animal consuming it (Case et al., 2000). If a dog and a horse are fed the same high-fiber diet, the horse will have a higher ME value due to its better ability to digest fiber compared with a dog. These same differences in digestion can be seen between dogs and cats, although not to the same extent as seen with an herbivore. Three possible methods can be used to determine the ME in a diet: direct determination using feeding trials and total collection methods; calculation from analyzed levels of protein, carbohydrates, and fats in the diet; and extrapolation of data collected from other species (Case et al., 2000).

Feeding Trials

Feeding trials using the species of concern are the most accurate method of determining the ME content of a food. However, this can be very time consuming and expensive and requires access to large numbers of test animals (Case et al., 2000). The Association of American Feed Control Officials (AAFCO), the government body that oversees pet food production, has certain requirements for feeding trials; in general, for a maintenance diet, they require a minimum of eight animals, at least 1 year of age, being fed the food in question for a minimum of 26 weeks. The food consumption is measured and recorded daily; individual body weights should be recorded at the beginning, weekly, and at the end; and a minimum database of bloodwork is required at the beginning and the end of the study. All animals are to be given a complete physical examination by a veterinarian at the beginning and the end of the study; they should be evaluated for general health and body and hair condition, with comments recorded. A number of animals, not to exceed 25%, may be removed for non–nutrition-related reasons only during the first two weeks of the study. A necropsy will be conducted on any animal that dies during the study. There are additional conditions for foods used during pregnancy, lactation, or growth (Hand et al., 2000). Manufacturers of some of the premium pet foods routinely measure the ME of their formulated pet foods and ingredients through the use of controlled feeding trials (Case et al., 2000). Feeding trials are obviously a time-consuming and expensive way to test ME in pet foods, but they are also the most accurate method and have the greatest potential to expose any deficiencies or excesses in a particular food.

Calculation Method

ME values can also be determined using the calculation method. This involves the use of mathematical formulas to estimate the ME of a food from its analyzed protein, carbohydrate, and fat contents. The formulas used for dog and cat diets have constants that account for fecal and urinary losses of energy (Case et al., 2000). The method does not account for digestibility or quality of ingredients; excesses or deficiencies may not be apparent.

When direct data are not available for particular food ingredients in a particular species, data from other species can be used. This is especially common with cat food ingredients. The species most often used for comparison is the pig. Although this method of estimating ME is not as accurate as direct measurement, data collected from swine experiments have been reported to correlate well with values from other species with simple stomachs (Case et al., 2000). The method used to attain AAFCO certification is required to be listed on the product label.

TABLE 1.1. **Examples of AAFCO certification claims.**

1.	Animal feeding trials using AAFCO procedures substantiate that _____ provides complete and balanced nutrition for maintenance.
2.	This product is formulated to meet the nutritional levels established by the AAFCO dog food profile for adult dogs.
3.	Animal feeding tests using AAFCO procedures substantiate that _____ provides complete and balanced nutrition for all life stages of cats.
4.	_____ is formulated to meet nutritional levels established by the AAFCO cat food nutrient profiles for growth and maintenance.

From Hand, M.S., Thatcher, C.D., Remillard, R.L., & Roudebush, P. 2000. Appendix J: 2000 AAFCO feeding protocols for dog and cat foods. In M.S. Hand, C.D. Thatcher, R.L. Remillard, & P. Roudebush (eds.), *Small animal clinical nutrition* (4th. ed., p. 1056). Marceline, MO: Walsworth Publishing for Mark Morris Institute.

Most companies that use feeding trials clearly state this; those that use calculation methods or extrapolation methods may be a little vague in how the certification is obtained.

Energy Density

Energy density of a pet food refers to the number of calories provided in a given weight or volume. In the United States, energy density is expressed in kilocalories (kcal) of ME per kilogram or pound of the food (Case et al., 2000). The energy density must be high enough for the animal to be able to consume sufficient food to meet its daily energy requirements. Energy density is the primary factor that determines the amount of food eaten each day (Case et al., 2000). The ability to maintain a normal body weight and growth rate provides the criteria used to determine the appropriate quantity of food to be fed.

Because energy intake determines total food intake, it is especially important that diets are properly balanced so that requirements for all other nutrients are met at the same time that energy requirements are met (Case et al., 2000). For this reason, it is more appropriate to express levels of energy-containing nutrients in a food in terms of ME rather than as a percentage of the food's weight (Case et al., 2000). Expressing nutrient content as units per 1,000 kcal of ME is called nutrient density (Case et al., 2000). Remember that fats contain almost three times the energy of proteins or carbohydrates and may be a small proportion of the diet's weight yet supply a majority of the calories. If you look only at weight, a diet may look low in fat but in fact may be just the opposite. When evaluating different diets, it is important to look at the caloric distribution of a food as well as nutrient density, rather than the percentage of the food's weight. This will allow you to compare foods of differing moisture or energy contents. This method is somewhat limited compared with the use of nutrient density, because caloric distribution considers only the energy-containing nutrients of the food. The AAFCO requires that the energy value of a pet food be expressed in kilocalories of ME (Case et al., 2000).

Excess energy intake in much more common in dogs and cats than is energy deficiency. Excessive energy intake has been shown to have several detrimental effects on dogs during growth, especially those of the large and giant breeds. Feeding growing puppies to attain maximal growth rate appears to be a significant contributing factor in the development of skeletal disorders such as osteochondrosis and hip dysplasia (Case et al., 2000). Excessive energy intake during growth also affects

TABLE 1.2. **Examples of nutrient density and caloric distribution.**

Dog food for growth, dry:
Calories (ME): 4,491 kcal/kg, 485 kcal/cup
Caloric distribution:
       Protein 29%
       Fat 46%
       Carbohydrate 25%

Dog food for maintenance, canned:
Calories (ME): 1,108 kcal/kg, 409 kcal/can
Caloric distribution:
       Protein 34%
       Fat 58%
       Carbohydrate 8%

Cat food for maintenance, dry:
Calories (ME): 4,490 kcal/kg, 459 kcal/cup
Caloric distribution:
       Protein 29%
       Fat 47%
       Carbohydrate 24%

Cat food, hairball formula, dry:
Calories (ME): 3,692 kcal/kg, 280 kcal/cup
Caloric distribution:
       Protein 30%
       Fat 29%
       Carbohydrate 41%

Therapeutic recovery diet, canned:
Calories (ME): 2,000 kcal/kg, 340 kcal/can
       2.14 kcal/ml—canine
       2.11 kcal/ml—feline
Caloric distribution:
       Protein 29%
       Fat 66%
       Carbohydrate 5%

From Roudebush, P., Dzanis, D.A., Debraekeleer, J., & Brown, R.G. 2000. Pet food labels. In M.S. Hand, C.D. Thatcher, R.I. Remillard, & P. Roudebush (eds.). *Small Animal clinical nutrition* (4th. ed., p. 155). Marceline, MO: Walsworth Publishing for Mark Morris Institute.

the total number of fat cells of an animal; if the animal overconsumes during the growth phase, this can contribute to the development of obesity later in life (Case et al., 2000). Obesity has been linked to the development of orthopedic problems later in life, as well as, increasing the incidence of diabetes, hyperlipidemia, pancreatitis, and heart failure. A study conducted by Nestle Purina demonstrated that by simply reducing the amount of food fed to a control group of Labradors by

TABLE 1.3. **Calculating nutrients as a percentage of metabolizable energy.**

Total calories in 100 g of food
Protein = (3.5 kcal/g) × grams in food
Fat = (8.5 kcal/g) × grams in food
Carbohydrate = (3.5 kcal/g) × grams in food
Total calories/100 g = protein calories + fat calories + carbohydrate calories

Percentage of ME contributed by each nutrient (caloric distribution)
Protein = [(protein calories/100 g)/(total calories/100 g)] × 100 = % ME
Fat = [(fat calories/100 g)/(total calories/100 g)] × 100 = % ME
Carbohydrate = [(carbohydrate calories/100 g)/(total calories)] × 100 = % ME

From Case, L.P., Carey, D.P., Hirakawa, D.A., & Daristotle, L. 2000. Fats. In *Canine and feline nutrition: A resource for companion animal professionals* (2nd. ed., pp. 19–22). St. Louis, MO: Mosby; and Gross, K.L., Wedekind, K.L., Cowell, C.S., Schoenherr, W.D., Jewell, D.E., Zicker, S.C., Debrakeller, J., & Frey, R.A. 2000. Nutrients. In M.S. Hand, C.D. Thatcher, R.L. Remillard, & P. Roudebush (eds.), *Small animal clinical nutrition* (4th. ed., pp. 59–66). Marceline, MO: Walsworth Publishing for Mark Morris Institute.

25%, they on average lived 1.5 years longer than their pair-mate and had less incidence of orthopedic problems, cancer, and metabolic diseases (Kealy et al., 2002).

Inadequate energy intake results in reduced growth rate and compromised development of young dogs and cats and in weight loss and muscle wasting in adult animals. In healthy animals, this is most commonly seen in hard-working dogs, pregnant or lactating females that are being fed a diet that is too low in energy density (Case et al., 2000). This can also be seen in sick animals that are either unable or unwilling to eat and in those whose disease process causes energy loss or increased energy use (Donoghue & Kronfeld, 1994).

References

Burger, I.H., & Thompson, A. 1994. Reading a pet food label. In J.M. Wills & K.W. Simpson (eds.), *The Waltham book of clinical nutrition of the dog and cat* (pp. 21–22). Terrytown, NY: Pergamon Press.

Case, L.P., Carey, D.P., Hirakawa, D.A., & Daristotle, L. 2000. Energy and water. In *Canine and feline nutrition: A resource for companion animal professionals* (2nd. ed., pp. 3–14). St. Louis, MO: Mosby.

Donoghue, S., & Kronfeld, D.S. 1994. Feeding hospitalized dogs and cats. In J.M. Wills & K.W. Simpson (eds.), *The Waltham book of clinical nutrition of the dog and cat* (p. 29). Oxford: Butterworth-Heinemann.

Gross, K.L., Wedekind, K.L., Cowell, C.S., Schoenherr, W.D., Jewell, D.E., Zicker, S.C., Debrakeller, J., & Frey, R.A. 2000. Nutrients. In M.S. Hand, C.D. Thatcher, R.L. Remillard, & P. Roudebush (eds.), *Small animal clinical nutrition* (4th. ed., pp. 21–36). Marceline, MO: Walsworth Publishing for Mark Morris Institute.

Hand, M.S., Thatcher, C.D., Remillard, R.L., & Roudebush, P. 2000. Appendix J: 2000 AAFCO feeding protocols for dog and cat foods. In M.S. Hand, C.D. Thatcher, R.L. Remillard, & P. Roudebush (eds.), *Small animal clinical nutrition* (4th. ed., p. 1056). Marceline, MO: Walsworth Publishing for Mark Morris Institute.

Kealy, R.D., Lawler, D.F., Ballam, J.M., Mantz, S.L., Biery, D.N., Greeley, E.H., Lust, G., Segre, M., Smith, G.K., & Stowe, H.D. 2002. Effects of diet restriction on life span and age-related changes in dogs. *Journal of the American Veterinary Medical Association, 220,* 1315–1320.

2

Water

Water is the single most important nutrient in terms of survivability. Animals can live for weeks without any food, using their own body fat and muscle for energy production, but a loss of only 10% of their body water results in death (Case et al., 2000; Gross et al., 2000; Wills, 1996).

Within the body, water functions as a solvent that facilitates cellular functions and as a transport medium for nutrients and the end-products of cellular metabolism. Water is able to absorb much of the heat that is generated during metabolic reactions with a minimal increase in temperature. Water also helps to transport heat away from the working organs through the blood (Case et al., 2000; Gross et al., 2000).

Water is an essential component in normal digestion because it is necessary for hydrolysis, the splitting of larger molecules into smaller ones through the addition of water (Case et al., 2000; Gross et al., 2000). Elimination of waste products through the kidneys also requires a large amount of water, which acts as both a solvent for the toxic metabolites and a carrier medium (Case et al., 2000; Gross et al., 2000).

Water is involved in regulating oncotic pressure, which helps the body to maintain its shape; one manifestation of loss of oncotic pressure is seen with dehydration in loss of skin elasticity. Water is found in all of the body fluids and helps to lubricate the joints and eyes, provides protective cushioning for the nervous system, and aids in gas exchange in respiration by keeping the alveoli moist and expanded (Gross et al., 2000).

Water accounts for the largest proportion of any of the nutrients in an animal's body, varying from 40% to 80% of the total amount. The percent of water varies with species, condition, and age (Gross et al., 2000). In general, lean body mass contains 70% to 80% water and 20% to 25% protein, with adipose tissue containing 10% to 15% water and 75% to 80% fat. The younger and leaner the animal is, the more water it contains. The fatter the animal, the lower is the animal's water content (Gross et al., 2000).

Water Loss

Water is lost in a number of ways. Obligatory loss from the kidneys is the minimum amount of water required by the body to rid itself of the daily load of urinary waste products. Facultative loss is the remaining portion of the urine that is excreted in response to the normal water reabsorption rate of the kidneys and to mechanisms responsible for maintaining proper water balance in the body. Fecal water accounts for a much smaller portion of the water lost (Case et al., 2000). A third route of water loss is through evaporation from the lungs during respiration. In dogs and cats, this water loss is very important for the regulation of normal body temperature during hot weather (Case et al., 2000).

Water Gains

Daily water consumption must compensate for these continual losses. The total water intake daily comes from three possible sources: water present in the food, metabolic water, and drinking water (Case et al., 2000).

The amount of water found in the diet depends on the type of food being fed; dry food can have moisture content as low as 7%, with some canned foods having a moisture content of as high as 84%. Within limits, increasing the water content of a food increases the diet's acceptability to the animal (Case et al., 2000).

Metabolic water is the water that is produced during oxidation of the energy-containing nutrients of the body. Oxygen combines with the hydrogen atoms contained in the carbohydrates, proteins, and fats in the food to produce water molecules (Case, 2003; Case et al., 2000). The metabolism of fat produces the greatest amount of metabolic water on a weight basis, and protein catabolism produces the smallest amount (Case et al., 2000). Metabolic water accounts for a fairly insignificant portion of the water intake, being only 5% to 10% of the daily total intake (Case et al., 2000).

The most significant source of water intake is voluntary drinking. Numerous factors can affect an animal's voluntary oral intake, including ambient temperature, type of diet being fed, level of exercise, physiologic state, and health (Case, 2003; Case et al., 2000). Water intake increases with an increase in ambient temperature and increasing exercise because of evaporative loss through the lungs due to panting to cool the body. The amount of food being fed can also affect water intake: as the calories increase, so does the amount of waste products that the body needs to get rid of, increasing the amount of urine produced. If this increase in calories results in weight gain, there will also be an increased loss due to panting to help with thermoregulation (Case, 2003; Case et al., 2000).

Voluntary Oral Intake

The type of diet being fed and the composition can dramatically affect voluntary oral intake of water. A study on dogs found that when the test animals were fed a diet containing 73% moisture, they obtained only 38% of their daily water needs from drinking water. When they were abruptly switched to a diet containing only 7% water, voluntary oral intake immediately increased to 95% or more of the total daily intake (Case et al., 2000). When cats are fed only canned food, their voluntary oral intake is likewise very low; in fact, when cats are fed a food with very high water content, they can maintain normal water balance with no additional drinking water (Case, 2003). This can be seen with liquid or gruel recovery diets, as well as some commercial canned diets with a high amount of sauce.

Water requirements are related to maintaining appropriate water balance in the animal. Dogs and cats meet the majority of their water requirements through water included in food and voluntary oral intake. As a general guideline, the daily water requirement, expressed in milliliters per day, for dogs and cats is roughly equivalent to the daily energy requirement (DER) in kcal/day. For dogs this is 1.6 multiplied by the resting energy requirement (RER); for cats, 1.2 multiplied by RER (Gross et al., 2000).

Domestic cats, which are descendents of desert animals, normally form more concentrated urine than do dogs. Water requirements for cats may be less than those for dogs (Case, 2003; Gross et al., 2000). Dogs will show thirst and drink voluntarily when body water decreases by 4% or less; cats do not voluntarily drink until they lose as much as 8% of their body water. In addition, cats that are fed dry food diets will typically consume less water per day than those fed canned food diets (Case, 2003).

If fresh, palatable, clean water is available and proper amounts of a balance diet are being fed, most dogs and cats are able to accurately self-regulate their water balance through voluntary oral intake (Case, 2003; Case et al., 2000; Gross et al., 2000).

References

Case, L.P. 2003. The cat as an obligate carnivore. In *The cat: Its behavior, nutrition and health* (pp. 295–297). Ames, IA: Iowa State Press.

Case, L.P., Carey, D.P., Hirakawa, D.A., & Daristotle, L. 2000. Energy and water. In *Canine and feline nutrition: A resource for companion animal professionals* (2nd. ed., pp. 3–14). St. Louis, MO: Mosby.

Gross, K.L., Wedekind, K.L., Cowell, C.S., Schoenherr, W.D., Jewell, D.E., Zicker, S.C., Debrakeller, J., & Frey, R.A. 2000. Nutrients. In M.S. Hand, C.D. Thatcher, R.L. Remillard, & P. Roudebush (eds.), *Small animal clinical nutrition* (4th. ed., pp. 21–36). Marceline, MO: Walsworth Publishing for Mark Morris Institute.

Wills, J.M. 1996. Basic principles of nutrition and feeding. In N.C. Kelly & J.M. Wills (eds.), *Manual of companion animal nutrition and feeding* (pp. 14–15). Ames, IA: Iowa State Press.

3

Carbohydrates

Carbohydrates are the major energy-containing parts of plants, making up between 60% and 90% of their dry-matter weight (Case et al., 2000). This class of nutrients is made up of the elements carbon, hydrogen, and oxygen. Carbohydrates are classified as monosaccharides, disaccharides, oligosaccharides, or polysaccharides and have the general formula of $(CH_2O)n$ (Case et al., 2000; Gross et al., 2000). Hydrogen and oxygen are usually present in the same ratio as that found in water (H_2O), giving rise to the name carbohydrate, or hydrated carbon (Price et al., 1993).

Carbohydrates act primarily as an energy source, but they may also be converted into body fat and stored, or serve as starting materials for the metabolism of other compounds (Price et al., 1993).

Monosaccharides

Monosaccharides are also called simple sugars, and they are the simplest form of carbohydrates, being composed of sugar units containing between three and seven carbon atoms (Case et al., 2000; Gross et al., 2000). The chief monosaccharides are glucose, fructose (fruit sugar), and galactose (milk sugar) (Case et al., 2000; Gross et al., 2000). Monosaccharides can combine with one another to form polymers, and these can be enormous molecules containing many thousands of individual monosaccharide units (Price et al., 1993).

Glucose is a moderately sweet simple sugar found in commercially prepared corn syrup and sweet fruits such as grapes and berries. It is also the chief end-product of starch digestion and glycogen hydrolysis in the body. Glucose is the form of carbohydrate found circulating in the bloodstream and is the primary form of carbohydrate used by the body's cells for energy (Case et al., 2000).

Fructose, commonly called fruit sugar, is a very sweet sugar found in honey, ripe fruits, and some vegetables. It is also formed from the digestion or hydrolysis of the disaccharide sucrose (Case et al., 2000).

Galactose is not found in a free form in foods. However, it makes up 50% of the disaccharide lactose, which is found in the milk of all mammals (Case et al., 2000).

Disaccharides

Disaccharides are made up of two monosaccharide units linked together. Lactose, the sugar found in mammalian milk, contains a molecule of glucose and a molecule of galactose. This is the only carbohydrate of animal origin (Case et al., 2000; Gross et al., 2000). Lactose intolerance, as seen in some adult animals, is caused by a deficiency of beta-galactosidase. This deficiency prevents the glucose and galactose molecules from separating, making this a nondigestible carbohydrate (Price et al., 1993). Sucrose, commonly called table sugar, contains a molecule of glucose linked to a molecule of fructose. This is the most common sugar found in plants (Case et al., 2000).

Oligosaccharides

Oligosaccharides are carbohydrates made up of 3 to 10 monosaccharide units. These units may be the same or a mix of different monosaccharides. They are often difficult to digest and, if found in quantity, as with some plant materials, may be associated with gastrointestinal disturbances or flatulence (Price et al., 1993). Oligosaccharides that contain fructose are called fructooligosaccharides (FOSs) (Gross et al., 2000). FOSs in the diet improve intestinal flora, increase nitrogen digestion and retention, improve stool quality, and reduce fecal odors (Case et al., 2000).

Polysaccharides

Polysaccharides consist of many thousands of monosaccharide units. They are found widely in plants, being used for cell wall material (cellulose) and energy storage (starch for plants and glycogen for animals) (Case et al., 2000; Price et al., 1993). Cereal grains such as corn, wheat, sorghum, barley, and rice are the major ingredients in pet foods that provide starch (Case et al., 2000). Complex carbohydrates of plant origin other than starch are referred to as dietary fiber, or nonstarch polysaccharides (Table 3.1). These include cellulose, hemicellulose, pectin, and the plant gums and mucilages (Case et al., 2000; Price et al., 1993). Plant fiber differs from starch and glycogen in that its monosaccharide units have a different bonding configuration (beta instead of alpha bonds). These bonds resist digestion by the gastrointestinal enzymes, making them unavailable for absorption in the small intestine (Case et al., 2000).

Certain microbes found in the large intestine of dogs and cats are able to break down fiber to varying degrees, even though the animal themselves are unable to break down the fiber (Case et al., 2000). This bacterial fermentation produces short-chain fatty acids (SCFAs) and other end-products. The SCFAs that are produced in the greatest numbers are acetate, propionate, and butyrate (Case et al., 2000).) These SCFAs are a significant energy source for the enterocytes and colonocytes of the large intestine (Case et al., 2000). Fiber in the diet also functions as an aid in the proper functioning of the gastrointestinal tract and as a dietary diluent that decreases the total energy density of the diet (Case et al., 2000).

Glycosaminoglycans are complex polysaccharides associated with proteins. They form integral parts of the interstitial fluid, cartilage, skin, and tendons. The primary glycosaminoglycans are chondroitin sulfate and hyaluronic acid (Gross et al., 2000).

TABLE 3.1. **Dietary fiber fermentation in dogs' chart.**

Fiber type	Solubility	Fermentability
Beet pulp	Low	Moderate
Cellulose	Low	Low
Rice bran	Low	Moderate
Gum arabic	High	Moderate
Pectin	Low	High
Carboxymethylcellulose	High	Low
Methylcellulose	High	Low
Cabbage fiber	Low	High
Guar gum	High	High
Locust bean gum	High	Low
Xanthan gum	High	Moderate

From Case, L.P., Carey, D.P., Hirakawa, D.A., & Daristotle, L. 2000. Carbohydates. In *Canine and feline nutrition: A resource for companion animal professionals* (2nd. ed., pp. 15–18). St. Louis, MO: Mosby.

Carbohydrate Functions

Carbohydrates have several functions in the body. The monosaccharide glucose is an important energy source for many tissues. A constant supply of glucose is necessary for the proper functioning of the central nervous system (CNS), and the glycogen present in the heart muscle is an important emergency energy source for the heart (Case et al., 2000). Glycogen in the liver and muscle can be hydrolyzed to supply additional energy to the cells when circulating glucose is low. Carbohydrates also supply carbon skeletons for the formation of nonessential amino acids and is needed for the synthesis of other essential body compounds such as glucuronic acid, heparin, chondroitin sulfate, the immunopolysaccharides, deoxyribonucleic acid (DNA), and ribonucleic acid (RNA) (Case et al., 2000). When joined with proteins or lipids, some carbohydrates also become important structural components in the body's tissues (Case et al., 2000). When metabolized for energy to carbon dioxide and water, they are a source of heat for the body (Gross et al., 2000). Finally, simple carbohydrates and starches consumed in excess of the body's needs are stored as glycogen or converted to fat (Gross et al., 2000).

Not only do carbohydrates provide energy to the body, digestible carbohydrates also have a protein-sparing effect. By providing enough carbohydrates to the body to meet its energy needs, protein is spared from being used for energy and is available for use in tissue repair and growth (Case et al., 2000; Gross et al., 2000). Conversely, if insufficient carbohydrates are available in the diet, protein will be used to meet energy needs, decreasing the amount available for tissue repair and growth (Case et al., 2000).

References

Case, L.P., Carey, D.P., Hirakawa, D.A., & Daristotle, L. 2000. Carbohydates. In *Canine and feline nutrition: A resource for companion animal professionals* (2nd. ed., pp. 15–18). St. Louis, MO: Mosby.

Gross, K.L., Wedekind, K.L., Cowell, C.S., Schoenherr, W.D., Jewell, D.E., Zicker, S.C., Debrakeller, J., & Frey, R.A. 2000. Nutrients. In M.S. Hand, C.D. Thatcher, R.L. Remillard, & P. Roudebush (eds.), *Small animal clinical nutrition* (4th. ed., pp. 36–48). Marceline, MO: Walsworth Publishing for Mark Morris Institute.

Price, C.J., Bedford, P.C.G., & Sutton, J.B. 1993. Nutrients and the requirements of dogs and cats. In J.W. Simpson, R.S. Anderson, & P.J. Markwell (eds.), *Clinical nutrition of the dog and cat* (pp. 20–22). Cambridge, MA: Blackwell Science.

4

Fats

Dietary fat is part of a group of compounds known as lipids that share the property of being insoluble in water (hydrophobic) but soluble in other organic solvents (Case et al., 2000; Gross et al., 2000). Lipids that are solid at room temperature are commonly called fats, and those that are liquid at room temperature are called oils (Gross et al., 2000).

Lipids can be further categorized into simple lipids, compound lipids, and derived lipids (Case et al., 2000). The simple lipids include triglycerides, which are the most common form of fat present in the diet, and waxes (Case et al., 2000). Triglycerides are made up of three fatty acids linked to one molecule of glycerol; the waxes contain a greater number of fatty acids linked to a long-chain alcohol molecule (Case et al., 2000). Compound lipids are composed of a lipid, such as a fatty acid, linked to a nonlipid compound. Lipoproteins, which carry fat in the blood stream, are a type of compound lipid. The derived lipids include sterol compounds, such as cholesterol and the fat-soluble vitamins A, D, E, and K (Case et al., 2000).

Triglycerides

Triglyceride is the most important fat in the diet, and it can be differentiated in foods according to the types of fatty acids that each triglyceride contains (Case et al., 2000). Fatty acids vary in carbon-chain length and may be saturated, monounsaturated, or polyunsaturated (Case et al., 2000). Saturated fatty acids contain no double bonds between the carbon atoms and are therefore "saturated" with hydrogen atoms. Monounsaturated fatty acids have one double bond, and polyunsaturated fatty acids (PUFAs) contain two or more double bonds (Case et al., 2000). In general, the triglycerides in animal fats contain a higher percentage of saturated fatty acids than do those in vegetable fats (Case et al., 2000).

Fats function in the body as a form of energy storage; major deposits of accumulated fat can be found under the skin (subcutaneous fat), around the vital organs, and in the membranes surrounding the intestines (Case et al., 2000; Gross et al., 2000). The deposits of fat also serve as insulators, protecting the body from heat loss, and as a protective layer around the vital organs to guard against physical injury (Case et al., 2000). Although animals have a limited capacity to store carbohydrates in the form of glycogen, they have an almost unlimited capacity to store surplus energy in the form of fat (Case et al., 2000). Fats also provide the body with essential fatty acids (EFAs) and provide a carrier for the fat-soluble vitamins (Case et al., 2000; Gross et al., 2000; Price et al., 1993).

Fat also has numerous metabolic and structural functions. Fat provides insulation around myelinated nerve fibers and aids in the transmission of nerve impulses. Phospholipids and glycolipids serve as structural components for cell membranes and participate in the transport of nutrients and metabolites across these membranes (Case et al., 2000).

Lipoproteins

Lipoproteins provide for the transport of fats through the bloodstream (Table 4.1). Cholesterol is used by the body to form the bile salts necessary for proper fat digestion and absorption, and it is also a precursor for the steroid hormones (Case et al., 2000). Along with other lipids, cholesterol forms a protective layer in the skin that prevents excessive water loss and the invasion of foreign substances (Case et al., 2000).

Of all of the nutrients, fat provides the most concentrated form of energy, being almost three times that of carbohydrates and proteins. The digestibility of fat is usually higher than that of carbohydrates and proteins (Case et al., 2000). This is especially important when the caloric density of a food must be increased—by increasing the fat, both the available calories and the digestibility of the food can be increased.

TABLE 4.1. **Lipoprotein classes.**

Lipoprotein	Acronym	Protein-to-lipid ratio
Chylomicron	CM	1:99
Very low-density lipoprotein	VLDL	10:90
Low-density lipoprotein	LDL	25:75
High-density lipoprotein	HDL	50:50

From Gross, K.L., Wedekind, K.L., Cowell, C.S., Schoenherr, W.D., Jewell, D.E., Zicker, S.C., Debrakeller, J., & Frey, R.A. 2000. Nutrients. In M.S. Hand, C.D. Thatcher, R.L. Remillard, & P. Roudebush (eds.), Small animal clinical nutrition (4th. ed., pp. 59–66). Marceline, MO: Walsworth Publishing for Mark Morris Institute.

Essential Fatty Acids

Dietary fat provides as source of the EFAs. These are generally recognized as linoleic acid, alpha-linolenic acid, and arachidonic acid. These are either omega 3 EFAs (alpha-linolenic acid) or omega 6 EFAs (linoleic acid and arachidonic acid) (Case et al., 2000; Gross et al., 2000; Price et al., 1993). The omega 3 and omega 6 fatty acids are essential because the body is unable to synthesize them. The omega 9 fatty acids and saturated fatty acids are able to be synthesized by the body and are seen as nonessential fatty acids (Gross et al., 2000). All of the EFAs are polyunsaturated fatty acids, with the position of the first double bond being denoted by the omega, counting from the terminal (methyl) end of the chain (Case et al., 2000; Gross et al., 2000). In most animals, gamma-linolenic acid and arachidonic acid can be synthesized from linoleic acid; if adequate linoleic acid is provided in the diet, there would be no dietary requirement for gamma-linolenic acid or arachidonic acid. The exception to this would be the cat, which requires a dietary source of arachidonic acid regardless of the amount of linoleic acid found in the diet (Case, 2003; Case et al., 2000). Unlike many other nutrients, instead of being broken down for digestion and use by the body, fats undergo elongation and desaturation (losing hydrogen atoms) for use in the body. Unsaturated fatty acids cannot be converted between families such as the omega 3 or omega 6 families, and monounsaturated and saturated fatty acids cannot be converted to EFAs (Gross et al., 2000).

As shown in Table 4.2, the first number for each of the fatty acids is the number of carbon atoms, the n designation indicates the number of double bonds, and the last number is the location of that double bond from the terminal methyl (CH_3) end.

TABLE 4.2. **Fatty acid structure.**

Saturated
Lauric acid (12:0)
$CH_3-CH_2-CH_2-CH_2-CH_2-CH_2-CH_2-CH_2-CH_2-CH_2-CH_2-COOH$

Monounsaturated
Palmitoleic acid (16:1n-7)
$CH_3-CH_2-CH_2-CH_2-CH_2-CH_2-CH=CH-CH_2-CH_2-CH_2-CH_2-CH_2-CH_2-CH_2-COOH$

Polyunsaturated
Linoleic acid (18:2n-6)
$CH_3-CH_2-CH_2-CH_2-CH_2-CH=CH-CH_2-CH=CH-CH_2-CH_2-CH_2-CH_2-CH_2-CH_2-CH_2-COOH$

Alpha-linolenic acid (18:3n-3)
$CH_3-CH_2-CH=CH-CH_2-CH=CH-CH_2-CH=CH-CH_2-CH_2-CH_2-CH_2-CH_2-CH_2-CH_2-COOH$

Arachidonic acid (20:4n-6)
$CH_3-CH_2-CH_2-CH_2-CH_2-CH=CH-CH_2-CH=CH-CH_2-CH=CH-CH_2-CH=CH-CH_2-CH_2-CH_2-COOH$

From Case, L.P., Carey, D.P., Hirakawa, D.A., & Daristotle, L. 2000. Fats. In *Canine and feline nutrition: A resource for companion animal professionals* (2nd. ed., pp. 19–22). St. Louis, MO: Mosby; and Gross, K.L., Wedekind, K.L., Cowell, C.S., Schoenherr, W.D., Jewell, D.E., Zicker, S.C., Debrakeller, J., & Frey, R.A. 2000. Nutrients. In M.S. Hand, C.D. Thatcher, R.L. Remillard, & P. Roudebush (eds.), *Small animal clinical nutrition* (4th. ed., pp. 59–66). Marceline, MO: Walsworth Publishing for Mark Morris Institute.

The best sources for linoleic acid (omega 6 family) are vegetable oils such as corn, soybean, and safflower oils. Pork fat and poultry fat also contain appreciable amounts of linoleic acid, but beef fat and butter fat contain very little (Case et al., 2000). Arachidonic acid (omega 3 family) can be found only in animal fats; this is especially important in cat diets. Because of the requirement for arachidonic acid, cats cannot be fed a balanced vegetarian diet, as the only source of arachidonic acid is animal fats (Case, 2003). Some fish oils are rich in arachidonic acid, and arachidonic acid is found in small amounts in poultry and pork fat (Case et al., 2000).

Omega 6 fatty acids have functionally distinct effects compared with those of the omega 3 family (Gross et al., 2000). Adding arachidonic acid to food where it was previously absent increases food efficiency and enhances skin condition by reducing water loss through the skin (Gross et al., 2000). This causes a shinier, glossier coat with less skin flaking. Eicosanoids (a product of any of the omega EFA families) that are produced from the omega 3 family are less immunologically stimulating than those from the omega 6 or 9 families. This means that they have less potential to produce an inflammatory reaction in the body (Gross et al., 2000). This is important in situations where decreasing the inflammatory response is desired, such as before and after surgery, after trauma, for burns, for injury or some types of cancer, or assisting in the control of dermatitis, arthritis, inflammatory bowel disease, and colitis (Gross et al., 2000). Adjusting the omega 3–to–omega 6 fatty acid ratio in therapeutic diets can assist in decreasing these responses.

Lipids are also essential for the absorption of the fat-soluble vitamins A, D, E, and K. The type of fat is not specific (Gross et al., 2000).

Fatty acid deficiencies in the diet impair wound healing, cause a dry lusterless coat and scaly skin, and change the lipid film on the skin, which can predispose the animal to skin infections. With an inadequate amount of fats, the fat-soluble vitamins are also not properly absorbed and deficiencies in these can be seen (Gross et al., 2000).

Most important for animals, fats improve the palatability and texture of the diets being fed (Case et al., 2000; Gross et al., 2000). The problem with this would be as the fat content of the diet increases, so does the caloric density and palatability; this can easily lead to overconsumption of the diet, which in turn leads to obesity.

References

Case, L.P. 2003. The cat as an obligate carnivore. In *The cat: Its behavior, nutrition and health* (pp. 295–297). Ames, IA: Iowa State Press.

Case, L.P., Carey, D.P., Hirakawa, D.A., & Daristotle, L. 2000. Fats. In *Canine and feline nutrition: A resource for companion animal professionals* (2nd. ed., pp. 19–22). St. Louis, MO: Mosby.

Gross, K.L., Wedekind, K.L., Cowell, C.S., Schoenherr, W.D., Jewell, D.E., Zicker, S.C., Debrakeller, J., & Frey, R.A. 2000. Nutrients. In M.S. Hand, C.D. Thatcher, R.L. Remillard, & P. Roudebush (eds.), *Small animal clinical nutrition* (4th. ed., pp. 59–66). Marceline, MO: Walsworth Publishing for Mark Morris Institute.

Price, C.J., Bedford, P.C.G., & Sutton, J.B. 1993. Nutrients and the requirements of dogs and cats. In J.W. Simpson, R.S. Anderson, & P.J. Markwell (eds.), *Clinical nutrition of the dog and cat* (pp. 22–23). Cambridge, MA: Blackwell Science.

5

Protein and Amino Acids

Proteins are large, complex molecules composed of hundreds to thousands of amino acids. These amino acids are composed of carbon, hydrogen, oxygen, nitrogen, and sometimes sulfur and phosphorus atoms (Case, 2003; Case et al., 2000; Gross et al., 2000). Although hundreds of amino acids exist in nature, only 20 are commonly found as protein components (Gross et al., 2000). Proteins are linear polymers of amino acids in which the amino group of one amino acid and the carboxyl group of another amino acid are joined together through a peptide bond. Amino acids joined together are called peptides, two bonded together are a dipeptide, three bonded together are a tripeptide, and more than three bonded together are a polypeptide (Gross et al., 2000). Once hydrolysis begins in the body, simple proteins yield only amino acids or their derivatives (Case et al., 2000). Proteins can also become bonded to other molecules; this yields a useful basis for simple classification (Price, Bedford, & Sutton, 1993).

Simple proteins give raise to their basic amino acids units only. Examples include the following:

- Albumins are globular proteins found in egg white, blood plasma, and milk.
- Collagens are fibrous proteins present in connective tissue and are converted to gelatin on prolonged boiling.
- Elastins are fibrous elastic proteins found in artery walls and skin (Price et al., 1993).

Conjugated proteins give raise to other distinctive substances in addition to amino acids:

- Glycoproteins contain carbohydrates, as seen with mucus.
- Lipoproteins contain lipid.
- Phosphoproteins contain a phosphorus group such as casein in milk.
- Chromoproteins contain a pigment group such as heme in hemoglobin.
- Nucleoproteins combine proteins and nucleic acids, as with DNA and RNA (Case et al., 2000; Gross et al., 2000; Price et al., 1993).

Protein is required in the diet to provide a source of amino acids to build, repair, and replace body proteins. They also supply nitrogen for the synthesis of the nonessential amino acids and other nitrogen-containing compounds (Case, 2003). Amino acids are divided into two groups: nonessential and essential (Table 5.1) (Case et al., 2000). The distinction between these two groups is that the essential amino acids must be included in the diet, while the nonessential amino acids can be synthesized by the body from other precursors at a rate sufficient to meet physiologic needs (Case et al., 2000).

Some proteins are conditionally essential, in that they are required in amounts exceeding the body's ability to produce them at times, usually during certain physiologic or disease conditions (Gross et al., 2000).

TABLE 5.1. Essential and nonessential amino acids for dogs and cats.

Essential amino acids	Nonessential amino acids
Arginine	Alanine
Histidine	Asparagine
Isoleucine	Aspartate
Leucine	Cysteine
Lysine	Glutamate
Methionine	Glutamine
Phenylalanine	Glycine
Taurine (cats only)	Hydroxylysine
Tryptophan	Hydrosyproline
Threonine	Proline
Valine	Serine
	Tyrosine

From Case, L.P., Carey, D.P., Hirakawa, D.A., & Daristotle, L. 2000. Proteins and amino acids. In *Canine and feline nutrition: A resource for companion animal professionals* (2nd. ed., pp. 23–28). St. Louis, MO: Mosby.

Functions of Proteins

Proteins in the body have numerous functions. They are the major structural components of hair, feathers, skin, nails, tendons, ligaments, and cartilage (Case et al., 2000). Contractile proteins such as myosin and actin are involved in regulating muscle action. All of the enzymes that catalyze the body's essential metabolic reactions and are essential for nutrient digestion and assimilation are also protein molecules (Case et al., 2000). Many hormones that control the homeostatic mechanisms of various body systems are composed of protein such as insulin and glucagon, both of which are involved in control of normal blood sugar levels. Proteins found in the blood act as important carrier substances, including hemoglobin to carry oxygen between the lungs and the cells and transferrin to carry iron (Case et al., 2000). Plasma proteins are also involved in maintenance of the acid-base balance. Finally, proteins are involved in the body's immune system to make the antibodies that provide resistance to disease (Case et al., 2000).

The cat has the highest overall protein requirement of any other mammal, including the dog (Case, 2003). This is not due to a higher requirement for essential amino acids, but rather because of some nitrogen catabolic enzymes in the liver of the cat that are permanently set to handle a high level of dietary protein; their activity is not modified even when the cat is receiving a low-protein diet (Price et al., 1993). Cats also lack the ability to conserve nitrogen from the body's general nitrogen pool. The inflexibility of liver enzyme activity and fixed high rate of catabolic activity basically obligate cats to consume a high-protein diet (Case, 2003).

All proteins in the body are in a constant state of renewal and degradation. Although tissues vary in their rate of turnover, all protein molecules in the body are eventually catabolized and replaced (Case, 2003; Case et al., 2000; Gross et al., 2000; Price et al., 1993). During periods of growth or reproduction, additional protein is needed for the creation of new tissue. A regular supply of protein and nitrogen is necessary to maintain normal metabolic processes and to provide for tissue maintenance and growth. The body does have the ability to synthesize new proteins from amino acids, provided that all of the necessary amino acids are available to the tissue cells (Case et al., 2000). A high rate of protein synthesis occurs in the production of red and white blood cells, epithelial cells of the skin, and those lining the gastrointestinal tract and the pancreas (Gross et al., 2000). Muscle protein composes nearly 50% of the total body protein but accounts for only 30% of the new protein synthesized. Visceral and organ proteins compose a smaller portion of the total body protein but account for 50% of the new proteins synthesized (Gross et al., 2000). Rates of protein synthesis and degradation for any particular protein can change under different physiologic conditions (Gross et al., 2000).

Dietary Protein

The body does not care where the amino acids come from for its use—whether they are synthesized by the body, supplied in the diet as single amino acids, or supplied as intact proteins. Because of this, it can accurately be said that the body does not have a "protein requirement" but rather an amino acid requirement (Case et al., 2000). Absorbed amino acids and small dipeptides and tripeptides are reassembled into "new" proteins by the liver and other tissues in the body (Gross et al., 2000). After absorption, the amino acids go toward tissue synthesis, especially muscles and liver; synthesis of enzymes, albumin, hormones, and other nitrogen-containing compounds; and deamination (removal of the amine group) and use of the remaining carbon skeletons for energy (Gross et al., 2000).

Proteins in the diet serve several functions. They provide the essential amino acids (which in turn are used for synthesis of protein in the growth and repair of tissue), and they are the body's primary source of nitrogen (Case et al., 2000). Nitrogen is essential for the synthesis of the nonessential amino acids and other nitrogen-containing compounds such as nucleic acids and certain neurotransmitter substances. Amino acids in the diet can also be metabolized for energy (Case et al., 2000). The gross energy of amino acids, once fecal and urinary losses are accounted for, are approximately the same as that of carbohydrates, 3.5 kcal/g (Case et al., 2000). Because animals are unable to store excess amino acids, surplus amounts either are used directly for energy or are converted to glycogen or fat for energy storage (Case et al., 2000).

Structural proteins in all tissues, especially in muscle, liver, and serum albumin, can be considered as amino acid stores (Gross et al., 2000). Muscle stores represent the largest reserve from which amino acids can be drawn in times of need, although too much loss of body protein can impair muscle function (Gross et al., 2000). Proteins in the diet also serve as an important source of taste: as the protein content of the diet increases, so do its palatability and acceptability (Case et al., 2000).

The degree to which a dog or cat is able to use the protein in the diet as a source of amino acids and nitrogen is affected by both the digestibility and the quality of the protein (Case et al., 2000). Proteins that are highly digestible and contain all of the essential amino acids in their proper proportions relative to the animal's needs are considered high-quality proteins. Those that are either low in digestibility or limiting in one or more of the essential amino acids are of lower quality (Case et al., 2000). The higher the quality of the protein in the diet, the less quantity will be needed by the animal to meet all of its essential amino acid needs (Case et al., 2000).

Protein Quality

The chemical score is an index that involves comparing the amino acid profile of a given protein with the amino acid profile of a reference of very high quality. Egg protein is typically used as the reference protein and is given a chemical score of 100. The essential amino acid that is in greatest deficit in the test protein is called the limiting amino acid because it will limit the body's ability to use that protein (Case et al., 2000). The percentage of that amino acid present in the protein relative to the corresponding value in the reference protein determines the chemical score of the test protein (Case et al., 2000). The three amino acids in food proteins that are most often limiting are methionine, tryptophan, and lysine. Having a chemical score can be helpful information regarding the amino acid deficits of a protein source, but its value is based entirely on the level of the most limiting amino acid in the food and does not take into account the proportions of all of the remaining amino acids (Case et al., 2000).

Biologic value is defined as the percentage of absorbed protein that is retained by the body. It is a measure of the ability of the body to convert absorbed amino acids into body tissue (Case et al., 2000). One problem with using biologic value as a measurement of protein quality is that it does not account for protein digestibility. In theory, if a small portion of a very indigestible protein that is absorbed is used efficiently by the body, it could still have a very high biologic value (Case et al., 2000).

Multiple protein sources are often combined in pet foods to improve the overall quality and amino acid profile when foods are formulated. By combining proteins based on their relative amino acid excesses and deficiencies, a food can be formulated with a higher-quality protein profile. This method of improving protein quality is called protein complementation (Gross et al., 2000). Amino acid fortification is another method for improving the protein quality in foods. In this method, one or more amino acids are added to a food when the main source of

TABLE 5.2. **Protein quality of common pet food ingredients.**

Ingredient	Percent protein	Chemical score	Biologic value
Egg (dried)	45% to 49%	100	94
Casein	80%	58	80
Beef, pork, lamb, chicken	29%	69	74
Soybean meal	48%	47	73
Whole corn	8%	41	59
White rice	7%	43	65
Wheat	14%	43	65
Collagen	88%	0	0

From Gross, K.L., Wedekind, K.L., Cowell, C.S., et al. 2000. Nutrients. In M.S. Hand, C.D. Thatcher, R.L. Remillard, & P. Roudebush (eds.), *Small animal clinical nutrition* (4th. ed., pp. 48–59). Marceline, MO: Walsworth Publishing for Mark Morris Institute.

protein may be limiting. This is seen most commonly with methionine and lysine (Gross et al., 2000).

Taurine

Taurine is an essential amino acid that in most mammals can be synthesized from methionine and cysteine. It belongs to a separate group of amino acids, called amino-sulfonic acids, and does not form part of the polypeptide chains like the other amino acids (Case, 2003; Price et al., 1993). Cats have a very limited ability to synthesize taurine from other sulfur-containing amino acids and therefore have an increased dietary requirement for it (Case, 2003; Price et al., 1993).

Taurine is necessary for bile acid conjugation to aid in the digestion of fats and is necessary for normal retinal function and myocardial function (Case, 2003). Taurine is present only in animal tissues. Consumption of a diet containing high levels of plant products and cereal grains may not provide sufficient taurine, even if meat-based products are included in the diet (Case, 2003).

Taurine requirements for cats consuming canned foods are substantially higher than those for cats consuming dry foods (Case, 2003; Price et al., 1993). The heat used to process the canned foods can damage the protein in the diet and lead to the production of indigestible protein byproducts. These products are less digestible than untreated protein and travel to the large intestine, where they are fermented by intestinal microbes. These bacterial populations responsible for the fermentation also degrade taurine (Case, 2003). This ultimately increases the fecal loss of taurine for the cats fed canned food diets. As a substantial proportion of the taurine requirements of adult cats are to replace the taurine lost in the feces through bile loss, anything that increases this loss also increases their requirements (Case, 2003).

References

Case, L.P. 2003. The cat as an obligate carnivore. In *The cat: Its behavior, nutrition and health* (pp. 295–297). Ames, IA: Iowa State Press.

Case, L.P., Carey, D.P., Hirakawa, D.A., & Daristotle, L. 2000. Proteins and amino acids. In *Canine and feline nutrition: A resource for companion animal professionals* (2nd. ed., pp. 23–28). St. Louis, MO: Mosby.

Gross, K.L., Wedekind, K.L., Cowell, C.S., Schoenherr, W.D., Jewell, D.E., Zicker, S.C., Debrakeller, J., & Frey, R.A. 2000. Nutrients. In M.S. Hand, C.D. Thatcher, R.L. Remillard, & P. Roudebush (eds.), *Small animal clinical nutrition* (4th. ed., pp. 48–59). Marceline, MO: Walsworth Publishing for Mark Morris Institute.

Price, C.J., Bedford, P.C.G., & Sutton, J.B. 1993. Nutrients and the requirements of dogs and cats. In J.W. Simpson, R.S. Anderson, & P.J. Markwell (eds.), *Clinical nutrition of the dog and cat* (pp. 23–27). Cambridge, MA: Blackwell Science.

6

Vitamins

Vitamins are defined by their physical and physiologic characteristics. In order for a substance to be classified as a vitamin, it must have five basic characteristics: (1) it must be an organic compound different from fat, protein, and carbohydrate; (2) it must be a component of the diet; (3) it must be essential in minute amounts for normal physiologic function; (4) its absence must cause a deficiency syndrome; and (5) it must not be synthesized in quantities sufficient to support normal physiologic function (Gross et al., 2000). These definitions are important, because not every vitamin is essential for every species.

Vitamins are needed in minute quantities to function as essential enzymes, enzyme precursors, or coenzymes in many of the body's metabolic processes (Case et al., 2000; Gross et al., 2000). A general classification scheme for vitamins divides them into two groups: the fat-soluble vitamins, A, D, E, and K; and the water-soluble vitamins, C and the B-complex vitamin group (Case et al., 2000). Because of the differences in water solubility and chemical structure in vitamins, they are absorbed into the body through a variety of means (Gross et al., 2000). Fat-soluble vitamins require bile salts and fat to form micelles for absorption: they are then passively absorbed (usually in the duodenum and ileum) and transported with chylomicrons to the liver via the lymphatics system (Gross et al., 2000). Water-soluble vitamins are absorbed by way of active transport; some vitamins require a carrier protein as with B12 (cobalamin) and intrinsic factor, where others require a sodium-dependent, carrier-mediated absorption pump (Gross et al., 2000).

Fat-soluble vitamins can be stored in the body's lipid deposits, making them more resistant to deficiency, but are more likely to cause toxicity (Case et al., 2000; Gross et al., 2000). Water-soluble vitamins are depleted at a faster rate because of limited storage and are less likely to cause toxicity but more likely to become deficient (Case et al., 2000; Gross et al., 2000).

Vitamin requirements differ based on the life stage of the animal. Growing and reproducing animals are making new tissues and therefore require higher levels of vitamins, minerals, protein, and energy for optimal performance (Gross et al., 2000). As animals age, metabolic and physiologic changes may also increase the requirements for vitamins (Gross et al., 2000). Various disease conditions may also affect vitamin status. Prolonged starvation deprives animals of vitamins and other nutrients and depletes the vitamin stores. Polyuric diseases such as diabetes mellitus and chronic renal failure may increase the excretion of water-soluble vitamins. Additionally, certain drugs, mainly antibiotics, may decrease the intestinal microflora responsible for vitamin K synthesis, and diuretic therapy may increase excretion of water-soluble vitamins (Gross et al., 2000).

Synthetic and naturally made vitamins are used by the body in the same way, although they may have different availability (Gross et al., 2000). All commercial pet foods contain vitamin supplementation. It is very difficult to formulate a diet that meets all vitamin requirements entirely from ingredient sources. Because of these vitamin additions, it is usually unnecessary and perhaps unwise to supplement commercial foods with additional vitamin supplements (Gross et al., 2000). Supplementation may be necessary in light of certain diseases but should be part of a monitored long-term treatment plan (Gross et al., 2000).

Fat-Soluble Vitamins

Vitamin A

Plants do not contain vitamin A per se but instead contain a provitamin in the form of carotenes. Beta-carotene has the greatest vitamin A activity compared with the other carotenoids but has only half the potency of pure vitamin A (Gross et al., 2000). The carotenoids are the dark red pigments in plants that provide the deep yellow-orange color of many plants (Case et al., 2000). Vitamin A can also be found in some animal tissues, with highest concentrations found in the liver and fish liver oils, as well as milk and egg yolks (Case et al., 2000; Gross et al., 2000).

Vitamin A is absorbed almost exclusively as retinol into the lymphatic system with low-density lipoproteins and transported to the liver, where it is deposited mainly in the hepatocytes and parenchymal cells (Gross et al., 2000).

Vitamin A is necessary for normal functioning in vision, bone growth, reproduction, tooth development, and maintenance of epithelial tissue including the mucous membranes lining the respiratory and gastrointestinal tracts (Gross et al., 2000).

With vitamin A deficiencies, differentiation of new epithelial cells fails to occur, and normal epithelial cells are replaced with dysfunctional cells. Epithelial cells that do not function properly lead to lesions in the epithelium and increased susceptibility to infection (Gross et al., 2000). Normal spermatogenesis in males and normal estrous cycles in females are also dependent on vitamin A (Case et al., 2000). Without vitamin A, the rods in the eyes become increasingly sensitive to light changes, which eventually lead to night blindness (Case et al., 2000).

Vitamin A toxicities can result in skeletal malformation, spontaneous fractures, and internal hemorrhage (Gross et al., 2000). Other signs may include anorexia, slow growth, weight loss, skin thickening, increased blood clotting time, enteritis, congenital abnormalities, conjunctivitis, fatty infiltration of the liver, and reduced function of the liver and kidneys (Gross et al., 2000).

Unlike dogs and most other animals, cats require preformed vitamin A. They lack the intestinal enzyme necessary to convert beta-carotene to active vitamin A (Case et al., 2000; Gross et al., 2000; Price, Bedford, & Sutton, 1993). Preformed vitamin A can be found only in animal tissues (Case et al., 2000; Gross et al., 2000; Price et al., 1993).

Vitamin D

Vitamin D consists of a group of compounds that regulate calcium and phosphorus metabolism in the body. The two most important of these compounds are vitamin D2 (ergocalciferol) and vitamin D3 (cholecalciferol). Vitamin D2 is found primarily in harvested or injured plants, not in living plant tissue. Because of this, it is only of importance to herbivores (Case et al., 2000). Vitamin D3 is synthesized in the skin of animals when its precursor, 7-dehydrocholesterol, is exposed to ultraviolet light from the sun (Case et al., 2000). This form of vitamin D can be obtained either through synthesis in the skin or from consumption of animal products that contain cholecalciferol (Case et al., 2000).

Both ingested and endogenous vitamin D3 are stored in the liver, muscle, and fat tissue. Cholecalciferol is an inactive storage form of vitamin D. To become active, it must first be transported from the skin or intestines to the liver, where it is hydroxylated (an OH compound is added) to 25-hydroxycholecalciferol. This compound is then transported to the kidneys, where it is further converted to one of several metabolites, the most active form being called calcitriol (Case et al., 2000; Gross et al., 2000). Although inactive vitamin D is considered a vitamin, calcitriol is often classified as a hormone because it is produced by the body and because of its mechanism of action (Case et al., 2000).

The primary function of vitamin D is to enhance intestinal absorption, mobilization, retention, and bone deposition of calcium and phosphorus (Gross et al., 2000). In the intestines, vitamin D stimulates the synthesis of calcium-binding protein, which enhances absorption of dietary calcium and phosphorus (Case et al., 2000). Vitamin D also affects normal bone growth and calcification by acting with parathyroid hormone to mobilize calcium from the bone and by causing an increase in phosphate reabsorption in the kidneys. The net effect of vitamin D's actions in the intestines, bones, and kidneys is an increase in plasma calcium and phosphorus to the level that is necessary to allow for normal mineralization and remodeling of the bone (Case et al., 2000).

Signs of vitamin D deficiency are frequently seen with simultaneous deficiencies or imbalances of calcium and phosphorus. Clinical signs generally include rickets in young animals, enlarged costochondral junctions, osteomalacia and osteoporosis in adult animals, and decreased serum calcium and inorganic phosphorus concentrations (Gross et al., 2000).

Vitamin D toxicity is usually associated with increases in vitamin D3 rather than vitamin D2. Excessive intake can result in hypercalcemia, soft tissue calcification, and ultimately death (Case et al., 2000).

Marine fish and fish oils are the richest natural sources of vitamin D in foods but may pose a risk for toxicity. Researchers have found that moist foods generally contain higher levels of vitamin D than dry foods, and some moist foods exceeded the Association of American Feed Control Officials (AAFCO) maximal allowances (Gross et al., 2000). Other sources include fresh water fish and egg yolks. Beef, liver, and dairy products contain smaller amount of vitamin D. The most common synthetic sources of vitamin D in pet foods include deactivated animal sterol (cholecalciferol), vitamin D3 supplementation, deactivated plant sterol (ergocalciferol), and vitamin D2 supplementation (Gross et al., 2000). For most animals, exposure to direct sunlight for ultraviolet production of vitamin D is poor due to their living situations (primarily house pets), darkly pigmented skin, or thick hair coats (Case et al., 2000).

Vitamin E

Vitamin E is made up of a group of chemically related compounds called the tocopherols and tocotrienols (Case et al., 2000; Gross et al., 2000). Alpha tocopherol is the most active form of vitamin E in the body and is the compound most commonly found in pet foods. Unfortunately, this form is also the least potent in the form of an antioxidant in foodstuffs; delta tocopherol is the most potent antioxidant for foods but is also the least biologically active form (Gross et al., 2000). Because of this mix of activities, vitamin analyses of foodstuffs are not a reliable means of determining vitamin activity (Gross et al., 2000). Most foods add mixed tocopherols to cover all the bases: biologic activity and antioxidant activity.

Within the body, vitamin E is found in at least small amounts in almost all the tissues, with the liver able to store the largest amounts (Case et al., 2000).

Vitamin E is absorbed from the small intestine via nonsaturable, passive diffusion into the intestinal lacteals and is transported via the lymphatics to the general circulation (Gross et al., 2000). Absorption of vitamin E is enhanced by the simultaneous digestion and absorption of dietary fats. There is a very high correlation between tocopherol levels and the total lipid or cholesterol concentration in the serum (Gross et al., 2000). The vitamin is found in highest concentrations in membrane-rich cell fractions such as the mitochondria and microsomes (Gross et al., 2000).

The need for vitamin E in the diet is markedly influenced by dietary composition, with increased need seen with increased levels of polyunsaturated fatty acids (PUFAs) in the diet, oxidizing agents, vitamin A, carotenoids, and trace minerals. Decreased need is seen in increased levels of fat-soluble antioxidants, sulfur-containing amino acids, and selenium (Gross et al., 2000). The chief function of vitamin E in the diet is as a potent antioxidant; PUFAs that are present in the foods and in the lipid membranes of the body's cells are very vulnerable to oxidative damage. Vitamin E interrupts the oxidation of these fats by donating electrons to the free radicals that induce lipid perioxidation (Case et al., 2000). Vitamin E also protects vitamin A and sulfur-containing amino acids from oxidative damage (Case et al., 2000).

Vitamin E has a relationship with the trace mineral selenium. Selenium is a cofactor for the enzyme glutathione peroxidase, which functions to reduce the peroxides that are formed during the process of fatty acid oxidation. The inactivation of these peroxides by glutathione peroxidase protects the cell membrane from further oxidative damage

(Case et al., 2000; Gross et al., 2000; Price et al., 1993). By preventing the oxidation of cell-membrane fatty acids and the formation of peroxides, vitamin E spares selenium, whereas selenium creates a similar effect and is able to reduce the animal's vitamin E requirement (Case et al., 2000; Gross et al., 2000; Price et al., 1993).

Deficiencies in vitamin E are seen primarily in the neuromuscular, vascular, and reproductive systems, with most signs being attributed to membrane dysfunction as a result of oxidative damage and disruption of critical cellular processes (Gross et al., 2000). Clinical signs in dogs include degenerative skeletal muscle disease associated with muscle weakness, degeneration of testicular germinal epithelium, and impaired spermatogenesis and failure of gestation. In cats, deficiency signs include steatites, focal interstitial myocarditis, focal myositis of skeletal muscle, and periportal mononuclear infiltration of the liver (Gross et al., 2000).

Vitamin E is one of the least toxic vitamins; animals can apparently tolerate very high doses without adverse effects. However, at extremely high doses, antagonism with other fat-soluble vitamins may occur, resulting in impaired bone mineralization, reduced hepatic storage of vitamin A, and coagulopathies as a result of decreasing absorption of vitamins D, A, and K (Gross et al., 2000).

Vitamin E is synthesized only by plants, the richest sources being vegetable oils and, to a lesser extent, seeds and cereal grains. Tocopherol concentrations are highest in green leaves. Animal tissues tend to be low in vitamin E, with the highest levels being found in fatty tissues (Gross et al., 2000).

Vitamin K

Vitamin K comprises a group of compounds called the quinones. Vitamin K1 (phylloquinone) occurs naturally in green leafy plants, and vitamin K2 (menoquinone) is synthesized by bacteria in the large intestine (Case et al., 2000; Gross et al., 2000; Price et al., 1993). Vitamin K3 (menadione) is the most common form of synthetic vitamin K and has a vitamin activity two to three times higher than that of natural vitamin K1.

Vitamin K is required for normal blood clotting, as it is needed for the production of normal prothrombin (factor II) and for the synthesis of clotting factors VII, IX, and X in the liver (Case et al., 2000; Gross et al., 2000; Price et al., 1993). Vitamin K is also involved in the synthesis of osteocalcin, a protein that regulates the incorporation of calcium phosphates in growing bone (Gross et al., 2000).

Vitamin K is found in green leafy vegetables such as spinach, kale, cabbage, and cauliflower. In general, animal sources contain lower amounts of vitamin K, although liver, egg, alfalfa meal, oilseed meal, and certain fish meals are fairly good sources (Case et al., 2000; Gross et al., 2000). The synthesis of vitamin K by intestinal bacteria of dogs and cats can contribute at least a portion, if not all, of the daily requirements for these species (Case et al., 2000). Coprophagy increases vitamin K absorption in dogs (Gross et al., 2000).

Deficiency can occur with intestinal malabsorption diseases, ingestion of anticoagulants (mouse or rat poisons), destruction of the gut microflora by antibiotic therapy, and congenital defects (Gross et al., 2000). Vitamin K3 has lower lipid solubility and is the most effective form of vitamin K for cases of malabsorption, whereas vitamin K1 is the only form of vitamin K effective in anticoagulant poisonings (Gross et al., 2000). Deficiency can also be seen in cats being fed certain commercial foods containing high levels of salmon or tuna (Gross et al., 2000).

Toxicity has been reported only once and occurred secondary to warfarin (rodenticide) ingestion when vitamin K1 was given intravenously (Gross et al., 2000).

Water-Soluble Vitamins

B-Complex Vitamins

The B-complex vitamins are all water-soluble vitamins that were originally grouped together because of similar metabolic functions and occurrence in foods (Case et al., 2000). These nine vitamins act as coenzymes for specific cellular enzymes that are involved in energy metabolism and tissue synthesis (Case et al., 2000). Coenzymes are small organic molecules that must be present with an enzyme for a specific reaction to occur (Case et al., 2000). The vitamins thiamin (B1), riboflavin (B2), niacin, pyridoxine (B6), pantothenic acid, and biotin are all involved in the use of food for energy. Folic acid, cobalamin (B12), and choline are important for cell maintenance and growth and/or blood cell synthesis (Case et al., 2000; Gross et al., 2000).

Thiamin

Thiamin, also called vitamin B1, is a component of the coenzyme thiamine pyrophosphate, which plays an important role in carbohydrate metabolism (Gross et al., 2000; Case et al., 2000; Price et al., 1993). The thiamin requirement of an animal would be directly related to the carbohydrate content of the diet being fed (Case et al., 2000; Price et al., 1993).

Thiamin is hydrolyzed to free thiamin by intestinal phosphatases before absorption by intestinal cells. Absorption takes place primarily in the jejunum via an active, carrier-mediated transport system. The absorbed thiamin is transported in red blood cells and plasma, and tissues then take up the thiamin. The heart, liver, and kidneys have the highest concentrations of thiamin in the body (Gross et al., 2000).

A deficiency of thiamin results in an impairment of carbohydrate metabolism with accumulation of pyruvic and lactic acids within the body. This results in clinical signs related to the central nervous system because of the dependence of this system on a constant source of carbohydrate for energy (Case et al., 2000; Price et al., 1993).

Thiamin deficiencies can be seen with inadequate dietary intake or with high intake of foods containing thiamin antagonists. Thiaminases are found in high concentrations in raw fish, shellfish, bacteria, yeast, and fungi. Thiaminases are destroyed by cooking (Gross et al., 2000).

Thiamin can be readily found in many foods, with good sources being brewer's yeast, whole grain cereals, organ meats, and egg yolk. Thiamin is heat labile and is progressively destroyed by cooking (Case et al., 2000; Gross et al., 2000; Price et al., 1993).

Riboflavin

Riboflavin, vitamin B2, is the precursor to a group of enzymatic cofactors called flavins. Flavins linked to proteins are called flavoproteins (Gross et al., 2000). It is named for its yellow color (flavin) and because it contains the simple sugar D-ribose (Case et al., 2000). It is relatively stable to heat processing but is easily destroyed by exposure to light and irradiation (Case et al., 2000).

Riboflavin functions in the body as a component of two different coenzymes: flavin mononucleotide and flavin adenine dinucleotide (Case et al., 2000). Both of these coenzymes are required in oxidative enzyme systems that function to release energy from carbohydrates, fats, and proteins, as well as in several biosynthetic pathways (Case et al., 2000).

After absorption in the intestinal tract, about 50% of the riboflavin in the blood is bound to albumin, and the other half is bound to globulins (Gross et al., 2000). Additionally, microbial synthesis of riboflavin occurs in the large intestine of most species (Case et al., 2000). The amount synthesized is dependent on the carbohydrate content of the diet (Gross et al., 2000).

Deficiency in dogs and cats is uncommon, but signs of dermatitis, erythema, weight loss, cataracts, impaired reproduction, neurologic changes, and anorexia can be seen. Toxicity has not been reported in the dog or cat.

Because there appears to be little storage of riboflavin in the body, daily intake of this vitamin is critical (Gross et al., 2000). Good sources of riboflavin include dairy products, organ meats, muscle meats, eggs, green plants, and yeast. Cereal grains are poor sources of riboflavin (Gross et al., 2000).

Niacin

The term "niacin" includes both nicotinic acid and nicotinamide and is closely associated with riboflavin in cellular oxidation-reduction enzyme systems (Case et al., 2000; Price et al., 1993). After absorption in the intestine, niacin is rapidly converted by the body into nicotinamide, the metabolically active form of the vitamin (Case et al., 2000). Nicotinamide is then incorporated into two different coenzymes: nicotinamide adenine dinucleotide and nicotinamide adenine dinucleotide phosphate (Case et al., 2000; Price et al., 1993). These coenzymes function as hydrogen-transfer agents in several enzymatic pathways involved in the use of fat, carbohydrate, and protein (Case et al., 2000; Price et al., 1993). Most animals can also synthesize niacin as an end-product of metabolism of the essential amino acid tryptophan (Case et al., 2000; Gross et al., 2000).

Niacin is a fairly stable vitamin, and processing conditions may actually release some bound niacin, which increases availability (Gross et al., 2000). Niacin deficiency may occur when foods low in niacin and tryptophan are eaten, such as corn and other grains. This deficiency results in a condition called pellagra, or black tongue. Signs seen are dermatitis, diarrhea, dementia, and death. Clinical deficiency in dogs in not common because most commercial foods are adequately supplemented. However, cats, because they are not able to synthesize substantial amounts of niacin from tryptophan and require preformed niacin, can develop deficiencies when fed high-cereal diets (Gross et al., 2000).

Niacin can be found in a wide variety of foods, with the greatest levels being found in yeast, animal and fish by products, cereals, legumes, and oilseeds. Unfortunately, a large portion of the niacin found in many plant sources is in a bound form and unavailable for absorption. The niacin found in animal sources is primarily in the unbound, available form (Case et al., 2000; Gross et al., 2000).

Pyridoxine

Vitamin B6 comprises three different compounds: pyridoxine, pyridoxal and pyridoxamine. All three are convertible in the animal to the coenzyme pyridoxal 5'-phosphate, which is the biologically active form of the vitamin (Case et al., 2000; Gross et al., 2000; Price et al., 1993). Pyridoxine is involved in a wide range of enzyme systems, particularly associated with amino acid metabolism and to a lesser extent in the metabolism of glucose and fatty acids (Case et al., 2000; Gross et al., 2000; Price et al., 1993). Pyridoxal 5'-phosphate is also required for the synthesis of hemoglobin and the conversion of tryptophan to niacin (Case et al., 2000). The pyridoxine requirements in the diet vary based on the protein levels in the diet (Case et al., 2000).

All the forms of B6 are freely absorbed via passive diffusion in the small intestine (Gross et al., 2000). The predominant form found in the blood is pyridoxal phosphate, which is tightly bound to proteins (Gross et al., 2000). Only small amounts of vitamin B6 are stored in the body, with any excesses and products of metabolism being excreted in the urine (Gross et al., 2000).

Reduced growth, muscle weakness, neurologic signs, mild microcytic anemia, irreversible kidney lesions, and anorexia are all signs of pyridoxine deficiency. Oxalate crystalluria is also a notable sign of pyridoxine deficiency in cats (Gross et al., 2000).

The incidence of toxicity is apparently very low; the earliest detectable signs include ataxia and loss of small motor control.

Vitamin B6 is widely distributed in foods, occurring in the greatest concentrations in meats, whole grain products, vegetables, and nuts (Gross et al., 2000). Plant tissues contain mostly pyridoxine, whereas animal tissues contain mostly pyridoxal and pyridoxamine (Gross et al., 2000). Pyridoxine is far more stable than either of the other two forms; thus, processing loss is greatest in foods containing high amounts of animal tissue (Gross et al., 2000).

Pantothenic Acid

Pantothenic acid is derived from the Greek word *pantos* meaning "found everywhere," because this vitamin occurs in all body tissues and in all forms of living tissue (Case et al., 2000; Gross et al., 2000). Once absorbed, pantothenic acid is phosphorylated by adenosine triphosphate (ATP) to form acetyl-coenzyme A (Case et al., 2000; Gross et al., 2000; Price et al., 1993). This is one of the most important coenzymes and is involved in the metabolism of carbohydrates, fats, and some amino acids within the citric acid cycle (Case et al., 2000; Gross et al., 2000; Price et al., 1993).

Acetyl-coenzyme A and acyl carrier protein are the primary forms of pantothenic acid found in foods. Both forms are degraded to pantothenic acid in the small intestine in a series of steps. Absorption occurs via a sodium-dependent energy-requiring process. At high concentrations, simple diffusion occurs throughout the small intestine. Pantothenic acid is transported in the free acid form in plasma. Red blood cells, which carry most of the vitamin, contain primarily acetyl-coenzyme A (Gross et al., 2000).

Dogs with pantothenic acid deficiency have erratic appetites, depressed growth, fatty livers, decreased antibody response, and hypocholesterolemia and can progress to coma in later stages (Gross et al., 2000). Cats with pantothenic acid deficiencies can develop fatty livers and become emaciated. Pantothenic acid is generally regarded as nontoxic. No adverse reactions or clinical signs are seen other than gastric upset in animals consuming large quantities (Gross et al., 2000).

Pantothenic acid is found in virtually all foodstuffs, so a naturally occurring deficiency is unlikely (Case et al., 2000; Price et al., 1993). The most important sources are meats, especially liver and heart, egg yolk, dairy products, and legumes (Case et al., 2000; Gross et al., 2000).

Folic Acid

Folic acid is also known as vitamins B10 and B11 as well as pteroylglutamic acid (Gross et al., 2000; Price et al., 1993). This is a family name for a group of vitamins with related biologic activity. Other common names include folate, folates, and folacin (Gross et al., 2000). Folic acid requires enzymatic changes to form the active compound tetrahydrofolic acid; from this molecule, the folate coenzymes used in the body are made (Price et al., 1993).

Folic acid acts as a one-carbon methyl donor and acceptor molecule in intermediary metabolism (Case et al., 2000; Gross et al., 2000). An important role of folic acid is its involvement in the synthesis of thymidine, a component of deoxyribonucleic acid (DNA) (Case et al., 2000). Vitamin B12 is also closely paired with folic acid in the production of methionine from homocysteine (Gross et al., 2000).

Natural sources of folic acid undergo hydrolysis by intestinal enzymes and are absorbed by enterocytes. Folic acid must be in the reduced form (i.e., dihydro-, tetrahydro-) to participate in one-carbon metabolic reactions (Gross et al., 2000).

Folic acid is synthesized by bacteria in the intestine, and this largely meets the daily requirement of the animals under normal circumstances (Price et al., 1993). It is required daily in the diet, as no reserves are kept in the body (Gross et al., 2000). Naturally occurring deficiencies would be uncommon but could be seen with deficient diets and with intestinal disease (Price et al., 1993). Clinical signs of folate deficiency are poor weight gain, anemia, anorexia, low white blood cell count, glossitis, and decreased immune function. There have been no reported cases of folate toxicity (Gross et al., 2000).

Folic acid is found in green leafy vegetables, organ meats, and egg yolks. The vitamin is destroyed by heating, prolonged freezing, and during storage in water (Case et al., 2000; Gross et al., 2000).

Biotin

Biotin was originally known as the "bios" factor. It is a sulfur-containing vitamin that functions as a coenzyme in several carboxylation reactions (Case et al., 2000; Gross et al., 2000; Price et al., 1993). It acts as a carbon dioxide carrier in reactions in which carbon chains are lengthened, specifically in certain steps of fatty acid, nonessential amino acid, and purine synthesis. In its active form, it is always found covalently bound to a protein (apoprotein) (Gross et al., 2000).

After ingestion, biotin must be hydrolyzed from protein by the enzyme biotinidase to be absorbed by the intestine. After hydrolysis, free biotin is absorbed through the intestine and transported through the blood to the tissues. Bacteria in the intestines are also able to synthesize biotin for use by the body (Price et al., 1993).

Naturally occurring biotin deficiencies are very rare in dogs and cats. Feeding raw egg whites and oral antibiotic use are probably the two most common causes (Gross et al., 2000). Egg white contains a compound called avidin, which binds biotin and makes it unavailable for absorption by the body (Case et al., 2000; Gross et al., 2000). Cooking destroys avidin and allows the biotin in the egg to be used. Avidin can also prevent absorption of endogenously produced biotin by the intestinal bacteria (Price et al., 1993). Clinical signs of biotin deficiency include poor growth, dermatitis, lethargy, and neurologic abnormalities (Gross et al., 2000). Biotin toxicity has not been reported in dogs and cats (Gross et al., 2000).

The biotin requirement is thought to be met by two sources, diet and intestinal microbes, because mammalian tissue is unable to synthesize it (Gross et al., 2000). Biotin is widely found in many foods, but bioavailability varies greatly. Oilseeds, egg yolks, alfalfa meal, liver, and yeast are good sources of biotin. Marked losses of biotin can occur as a result of oxidation, canning, heat, and solvent extraction of foodstuffs (Case et al., 2000; Gross et al., 2000).

Cobalamin

Vitamin B12 is the only vitamin that contains a trace element, cobalt. Cobalamin is the largest and most complex of the B vitamins (Gross et al., 2000). When isolated from natural sources, it is usually found in the form of cyanocobalamin. When transformed to a metabolically active coenzyme, the cyano group is replaced by another chemical group attached to the cobalt group (Price et al., 1993).

Cobalamin and its metabolites are important in one-carbon metabolism during various biochemical reactions and are involved in fat and carbohydrate metabolism, as well as myelin synthesis (Case et al., 2000; Gross et al., 2000). The function of vitamin B12 is closely linked to that of folate (Case et al., 2000; Gross et al., 2000; Price et al., 1993).

Cobalamin absorption depends on dietary intake and adequate gastrointestinal tract function. In most animals, absorption of cobalamin from the diet is facilitated by a protein called intrinsic factor, which is produced in the intestine (Case et al., 2000; Gross et al., 2000). The absence of this factor can lead to vitamin B12 deficiency (Case et al., 2000; Gross et al., 2000).

Vitamin B12 deficiency is very rare but may result in poor growth and neuropathies. Because vitamin B12 is only made by microbes and found in animal tissues, a vegetarian diet may lead to deficiencies (Gross et al., 2000). Toxicities have not been found in dogs and cats other than those given excessive amounts parenterally (Gross et al., 2000).

Good sources of cobalamin include organ meats, fish, and dairy products. This vitamin is unique in that once it is absorbed from the diet, excess amounts can be stored by the body. The primary place of storage is the liver, although muscle, bone, and skin can also contain small amounts (Case et al., 2000).

Choline

Choline is classified as one of the B-complex vitamins, even though it does not entirely satisfy the strict definition of a vitamin (Gross et al., 2000). Choline, unlike the other B vitamins, can be synthesized in the liver from the amino acid serine. In this reaction, methionine acts as a methyl donor, with folic acid and cobalamin also being needed. It is required in much larger quantities by the body than the other B vitamins (Case et al., 2000; Gross et al., 2000). Because of this, even though it is an essential nutrient, not all animals require it as a dietary supplement. Choline also does not function as a coenzyme or cofactor, as do most other vitamins (Gross et al., 2000).

Choline functions as an integral part of cellular membranes as the phospholipid lecithin, to promote lipid transport as phosphatidylcholine, as a neurotransmitter as acetylcholine, and as a source of methyl groups for transmethylation reactions (Case et al., 2000; Gross et al., 2000; Price et al., 1993).

Choline is released from lecithin in the diet by digestive enzymes in the intestinal tract, and it is absorbed from the jejunum and ileum mainly by a carrier-mediated process. Once absorbed, choline is transported through the lymphatic system in the form of phosphatidylcholine bound to chylomicrons (Gross et al., 2000).

Because on its synthesis in the liver, its presence in many foods, and the ability of methionine to spare choline, dietary deficiencies of choline have not been reported in cats and dogs (Case et al., 2000).

Dietary sources include egg yolks, organ meats, legumes, dairy products, and whole grains (Case et al., 2000).

Vitamin C

Ascorbic acid can be synthesized from glucose by plants and most animals, including dogs and cats. Chemically, its structure is closely related to that of the monosaccharide sugars (Case et al., 2000; Gross et al., 2000). Vitamin C functions in the body as an antioxidant and free radical scavenger (Gross et al., 2000). Ascorbic acid is best known for its role in collagen synthesis, although it is also involved in drug, steroid, and tyrosine metabolism and electron transport in cells (Gross et al., 2000). It is necessary for synthesis of carnitine to act as a carrier for acyl groups across mitochondrial membranes (Gross et al., 2000). Larger doses may play an important role in immune function and protection against carcinogens (Gross et al., 2000). Ascorbic acid acts as a nitrate scavenger, thereby reducing nitrosamine-induced carcinogenesis.

Dogs and cats are able to synthesize adequate amounts of ascorbic acid; therefore, dietary amounts are absorbed via passive diffusion in the intestinal tract (Gross et al., 2000). Absorption efficiency is unusually high, about 80% to 90% (Gross et al., 2000). Vitamin C is transported in the plasma in association with albumin. It is found widely distributed in all body tissues, with the pituitary and adrenal glands having the highest concentrations (Gross et al., 2000).

Deficiency is unlikely due to dogs and cats being able to synthesize most, if not all, of their requirements (Case et al., 2000). Toxicity has not been seen in dogs and cats (Gross et al., 2000).

Sources of vitamin C include fruits, vegetables, and organ meats. The vitamin C content of most foods decreases dramatically during storage and processing, as it is easily destroyed by oxidative processes. Exposure to heat, light, alkalines, oxidative enzymes, and the minerals copper and iron can all increase losses of vitamin C activity (Case et al., 2000).

Vitamin-Like Substances

Carnitine

L-Carnitine is a natural compound found in all animal cells (Gross et al., 2000). Its primary function is to transport long-chain fatty acids across the inner mitochondrial membrane into the mitochondrial matrix for oxidation (Gross et al., 2000). It is synthesized primarily in the liver and stored in the skeletal and cardiac muscles (Case et al., 2000; Gross et al., 2000).

Lysine, methionine, ascorbic acid, ferrous ions, vitamin B6, and niacin are all important in L-carnitine metabolism; these nutrients are required substrates and cofactors for enzymes involved in biosynthesis (Gross et al., 2000).

Clinical signs of L-carnitine deficiency include chronic muscle weakness, fasting hypoglycemia, cardiomyopathy, and hepatomegaly (Gross et al., 2000). In many cases of deficiency, no clinical signs are seen (Gross et al., 2000).

Carotenoids

This is a group of pigments that exhibit vitamin-like activities. More than 600 different compounds are classified as carotenoids, but fewer than 20% can be metabolized into vitamin A (Gross et al., 2000). The carotenoids found in the greatest numbers in a variety of foods include beta-carotene, alpha-carotene, lutein, lycopene, beta-cryptoxanin, zeaxanthin, canxanthin, and astaxanthin (Gross et al., 2000).

Catotenoids are digested and absorbed into the body using bile salts. Carotenoids are incorporated into micelles, where they are absorbed by the small intestinal mucosa by way of passive diffusion (Gross et al., 2000). After transportation in chylomicrons in the lymphatic system, they are bound to lipoproteins and transported into the bloodstream (Gross et al., 2000).

Carotenoids have biologic activity beyond their vitamin A role. Carotenoids with nine or more double bonds function as antioxidants, and they also protect cell membranes by stabilizing the oxygen radicals produced (Gross et al., 2000).

Carotenoids are found abundantly in orange and green vegetables, highly pigmented fruits, and some species of fish (Gross et al., 2000).

Bioflavonoids

The bioflavonoids are another group of red, blue, and yellow pigments consisting of over 4,000 different compounds but not classified as carotenoids. Like the carotenoids, they also have vitamin-like activities (Gross et al., 2000).

Flavonoids are usually found naturally as glycosides linked to sugars. Mammalian enzymatic systems are unable to hydrolyze flavonoids, but the necessary enzymes are present in the gut microflora (Gross et al., 2000). After hydrolysis and absorption in the small intestines, flavonoids are bound in the liver.

The flavonoids have a sparing effect on vitamin C; they also have the ability to perform similar to vitamin C. Flavonoid reactions are involved in the antioxidant system for lipid and water environments.

Bioflavonoids are found most abundantly in the skins and peels of colored fruits and vegetables (Gross et al., 2000).

References

Case, L.P., Carey, D.P., Hirakawa, D.A., & Daristotle, L. 2000. Vitamins. In *Canine and feline nutrition: A resource for companion animal professionals* (2nd. ed., pp. 29–40). St. Louis, MO: Mosby.

Gross, K.L., Wedekind, K.L., Cowell, C.S., Schoenherr, W.D., Jewell, D.E., Zicker, S.C., Debrakeller, J., & Frey, R.A. 2000. Nutrients. In M.S. Hand, C.D. Thatcher, R.L. Remillard, & P. Roudebush (eds.), *Small animal clinical nutrition* (4th. ed., pp. 80–95). Marceline, MO: Walsworth Publishing for Mark Morris Institute.

Price, C.J., Bedford, P.C.G., & Sutton, J.B. 1993. Nutrients and the requirements of dogs and cats. In J.W. Simpson, R.S. Anderson, & P.J. Markwell (eds.), *Clinical nutrition of the dog and cat* (pp. 30–37). Cambridge, MA: Blackwell Science.

7

Minerals

Minerals are the inorganic portion of the diet. Some are required in large quantities because they form a major part of the body's structural components, whereas others are only required in small quantities for the chemical processes of metabolism (Price et al., 1993).

As with most other nutrients, problems with minerals in the diet are usually related more to excesses or imbalances due to interactions with other nutrients rather than to actual deficiencies in the diet (Case et al., 2000). Because of this, in a diet that is known to be nutritionally complete in its mineral content, further supplementation is at best wasteful and at worst dangerous to the health of the animal (Price et al., 1993).

More than 18 minerals are believed to be essential for mammals. By definition, macrominerals are required by the animal in the diet in percentage amounts, whereas microminerals are required at a parts-per-million (ppm) level (Gross et al., 2000).

Minerals are used by the body for structural components, as seen with calcium, phosphorus, and magnesium in bones and teeth; as portions of body fluids and tissues, as with the electrolytes sodium, potassium, phosphorus, calcium, and magnesium; and as catalysts/cofactors in enzyme and hormone systems, as seen with iodine and selenium (Gross et al., 2000).

Availability of minerals from the diet, as well as how effectively the mineral can be used by the individual animal, can be affected by a number of factors. These factors include the chemical form of the mineral, which affects solubility; the amounts and proportions of other dietary components that the mineral interacts with metabolically; the age, gender, and species of the animal; the intake of the mineral and the body's need (amount found in the body's stores); and environmental factors (Gross et al., 2000).

Meat-derived foods are considered a more available source of certain minerals than are plant-derived foods. The organic forms of minerals found in meats are often more available or as available as those from inorganic mineral supplements, while those found in plants are often less available (Gross et al., 2000). Meats, unlike plants, do not contain antinutritional factors, such as phytate, oxalate, goitrogens, and fibers. These all have the potential to reduce mineral availability in the diet (Gross et al., 2000). Also, different forms of minerals differ in availability based on what they are combined with; generally, sulfur and chloride forms have the best availability, followed by carbonates, with oxides being the most poorly available (Gross et al., 2000).

Macrominerals

Calcium

Calcium has two important functions within the body. It is necessary for the formation and maintenance of the skeleton and teeth, and it acts as an intracellular messenger that allows cells to respond to stimuli such as hormones and neurotransmitters (Gross et al., 2000).

Calcium serves two physiologic functions in bones—as structural material and as a storage site for calcium (Gross et al., 2000). The amount of calcium absorbed from the diet can range from 25% to 90%, depending on calcium status, the form of the calcium, and intake in the diet (Gross et al., 2000). The calcium found in blood, lymph, and other body fluids accounts for only about 1% of the total calcium in the body, with the remaining 99% found in the bones and teeth (Gross et al., 2000).

Calcium absorption by the body can be either active regulated by vitamin D, facilitated, or passive absorption. Regardless of how the calcium is absorbed, vitamin D is the most important regulator of calcium absorption (Gross et al., 2000).

Deficiencies are uncommon today in well-formulated pet foods. Calcium imbalances can occur as a result of poor feeding practices. Calcium deficiencies are most common when dogs and cats are fed "table scrap" diets or all-meat diets consisting primarily of muscle and organ meats (Case et al., 2000; Gross et al., 2000). This is a very low-calcium, high-phosphorus diet that can develop into nutritional secondary hyperparathyroidism. The low levels of dietary calcium stimulate the release of parathyroid hormone (PTH). PTH increases the resorption of calcium from the bone in an attempt to increase the serum calcium levels. Eventually, this can lead to significant bone loss with resultant pathologic fractures (Case et al., 2000; Gross et al., 2000). Calcium excesses are most commonly due to dietary supplementation, especially of large breed, fast-growing puppies. By oversupplementing the diet with calcium, deficiencies can be produced in other nutrients as well as potentially causing an increased incidence of osteochondritis dessecans (OCD), hypertrophic osteodystrophy (HOD), and Wobbler's syndrome, among others (Case et al., 2000; Gross et al., 2000).

A relative calcium deficiency can also be seen with eclampsia, although this is more of a problem of calcium homeostasis in the body (Case et al., 2000). Eclampsia is seen most often in small breed dogs and less frequently in cats (Case et al., 2000). This is usually seen 2 to 3 weeks after parturition and is caused by a failure of the mother's calcium regulatory system to maintain serum calcium levels when there is loss of calcium in the milk (Case et al., 2000). With subnormal calcium serum levels, seizures and tetany can be seen. Prognosis is good if treatment is started at an early stage (Case et al., 2000). Excess calcium supplementation to try to prevent this problem can actually exacerbate it. When calcium intake is high, the PTH level is low. As milk production increases, calcium is lost in the milk, normally; PTH would be stimulated to release calcium from the bone to maintain serum levels. The PTH is unable to respond quickly enough to prevent dangerously low serum levels from occurring in the mother (Case et al., 2000). The best course of preventative action is to feed a high-quality commercial diet that has been formulated for growing animals and gestation (Case et al., 2000).

Calcium can be found in meat meals because of their bone content, soybean meal, and flaxseed meal. Grains and meats without bones are poor sources of calcium. The most common supplements used in pet foods include calcium carbonate (limestone), calcium sulfate, calcium chloride, calcium phosphate, and bone meal (Gross et al., 2000).

Phosphorus

After calcium, phosphorus is the largest constituent found in bones and teeth. Phosphorus is a structural component of RNA and DNA, as well as energy-generating compounds such as adenosine triphosphate (ATP) and a part of the phospholipids found in cell membranes (Gross et al., 2000). These functions make it essential for cell growth and differentiation, energy use and transfer, fatty acid transport, and amino acid and protein formation (Gross et al., 2000).

Generally, phosphorus is more available from animal-based ingredients than from plant-based ingredients (Gross et al., 2000). Phosphorus found in meats is primarily in the organic form, whereas that found in plants is in the form of phytic acid, which is only about 30% available to monogastric animals (Gross et al., 2000). Phytic acid is a phosphorus-containing compound that can bind other minerals, including calcium, and make them unavailable for absorption (Case et al., 2000).

Regulation of phosphorus within the body involves the coordinated efforts of both the intestines and the kidneys. When dietary intake is low, intestinal absorption is highly efficient and the kidneys decrease urinary losses. When dietary intake is high, intestinal absorption decreases and urinary losses increase (Gross et al., 2000).

High levels of phosphorus can be found in meats, eggs, and milk products. The primary supplements used in pet foods include calcium phosphate, sodium phosphate, and phosphoric acid (Gross et al., 2000).

Magnesium

Magnesium in the third largest mineral constituent found in the body after calcium and phosphorus (Gross et al., 2000). It is involved in the metabolism of carbohydrates and lipids, as well as acting as a catalyst for a wide variety of enzymes. As a cation (a positively charged particle) in the intracellular fluid, magnesium is essential for the cellular metabolism of both carbohydrates and proteins. Protein synthesis also requires the presence of ionized magnesium (Case et al., 2000). Magnesium can be found in soft tissue and bone as well as the intracellular and extracellular fluids (Case et al., 2000). A number of dietary and physiologic factors can negatively affect magnesium absorption, including high levels of phosphorus, calcium, potassium, fat, and protein in the diet (Gross et al., 2000).

Magnesium homeostasis within the body is controlled primarily through the kidneys; because of this, certain drugs can cause increased renal excretion of magnesium. These would include diuretics, aminoglycosides, cisplatin, cyclosporine, amphotericin, and methotrexate (Gross et al., 2000).

A deficiency of magnesium in the diet results in signs of weakness, ataxia, with eventual progression to seizures. Naturally occurring magnesium deficiency is usually not seen in healthy dogs and cats (Case et al., 2000). Avoiding excess magnesium is recommended to prevent the formation of struvite crystals and stones in the urine (Gross et al., 2000).

In sick animals, magnesium deficiencies can be seen with gastrointestinal and kidney diseases (Gross et al., 2000).

Sources of magnesium in the diet include ingredients containing bone (bone meals), oilseeds (flaxseed and soybean meal), and unrefined grains and fiber sources (wheat bran, oat bran, and beet pulp). Common supplements found in pet foods are magnesium oxide and magnesium sulfate (Gross et al., 2000).

Sodium and Chloride

Sodium and chloride are the major electrolytes of the extracellular fluids and are important for maintaining osmotic pressure, regulating acid-base balance, and transmitting nerve impulses and muscle contractions (Case et al., 2000; Gross et al., 2000). Sodium ions must also be present in the intestinal lumen for absorption of sugars and amino acids (Gross et al., 2000). Calcium absorption and mobilization are affected by the presence of sodium, and the absorption of several vitamins (e.g., riboflavin, thiamin, and ascorbic acid) is sodium dependent (Gross et al., 2000).

Sodium and chloride are readily absorbed primarily from the small intestine, with excretion primarily in the urine, although small amounts can be in the feces and perspiration (Gross et al., 2000). In very low-sodium diets, the body has a remarkable ability to conserve sodium by excreting very low amounts in the urine (Gross et al., 2000).

Concentrations of sodium in the body are regulated by various hormones acting to maintain a constant sodium-to-potassium ratio in the extracellular fluid (Gross et al., 2000). Sodium requirements are influenced by reproductive status, lactation, rapid growth, and heat stress.

When consuming a diet with high levels of sodium, a secondary increase in water intake is seen, as well as an increase in urination with high salt excretion by the kidneys accompanying this (Case et al., 2000). Studies have indicated that dogs and cats are resistant to salt retention and hypertension when fed diets high in sodium compared with humans (Case et al., 2000).

Fish, eggs, dried whey, poultry byproduct meal, and soy isolate are all high in sodium and chloride (Gross et al., 2000). Typically, dietary supplements added to pet foods include salt, sodium phosphates, calcium chloride, choline chloride, potassium chloride, and sodium acetate (Gross et al., 2000).

Microminerals

Iron

Iron is present in several enzymes and other proteins responsible for oxygen activation, electron transport, and oxygen transport. Iron found in food exists primarily as heme iron present in hemoglobin and myoglobin and as nonheme iron found in grains and other plants (Gross et al., 2000). The amount of iron absorbed from food is dependent on the iron status of the body, the availability of dietary iron, and the amounts of heme and nonheme iron found in the food (Gross et al., 2000).

Iron is transported via plasma to the bone marrow, where it is used for hemoglobin synthesis (Gross et al., 2000). It is stored primarily as ferritin and hemosiderin in the liver, bone marrow, and spleen (Gross et al., 2000). Excretion of iron is limited, with only small amounts being found in the urine. The iron appearing in the feces is primarily unabsorbed iron, although it is continually lost in sweat, hair, and nails (Gross et al., 2000).

Excesses of iron in the diet should be avoided because of potential antagonism with other minerals, primarily copper and zinc (Gross et al., 2000). Chronic blood loss will eventually deplete iron stores and cause a microcytic, hypochromic anemia. This is seen most commonly with parasitic infections, both intestinal in the form of hookworms and external with fleas and ticks (Gross et al., 2000). Young animals are especially at risk due to their low iron stores and the low iron content in milk (Gross et al., 2000).

High levels of iron are found in most meats, especially organ meats; other sources include beet pulp, soymill run, and peanut hulls (Gross et al., 2000). Typical iron additives used in pet foods include ferrous sulfate, ferric chloride, ferrous fumarate, ferrous carbonate, and iron oxide (Gross et al., 2000). Iron oxide is not biologically available to dogs and cats but is added to foods to give it a "meaty red" color (Gross et al., 2000).

Zinc

Second only to iron, zinc is the most abundant micromineral found in the body. It is important for carbohydrate, lipid, protein, and nucleic acid metabolism. It is also necessary for the maintenance of normal skin integrity, taste, and immunologic functioning (Case et al., 2000; Gross et al., 2000).

Homeostasis is controlled through absorption and excretion. Absorption occurs primarily in the small intestine. This absorption is markedly affected by other dietary components (Gross et al., 2000). Phytate, found in many plants, decreases zinc absorption, whereas certain materials such as citrate, picolinate, EDTA, and amino acids such as histidine and glutamate increase zinc absorption (Gross et al., 2000). The liver is the primary organ involved with zinc metabolism. Storage of zinc is limited except in the bone. Stores increase only slightly when dietary levels increase (Gross et al., 2000).

Signs of zinc deficiency can be seen in animals fed high-cereal diets, due to the phytate found in them. This, in combination with calcium, forms an insoluble complex of phytate, calcium, and zinc (Gross et al., 2000). Deficiency can be seen even when zinc levels in the diet exceed recommended levels (Gross et al., 2000). The only reported cases of toxicity have been due to dietary indiscretion as seen with the eating of pennies, die-case nuts from animal carriers, and baby lotions containing zinc (Gross et al., 2000). Excesses in the diet can interfere with absorption of other minerals, primarily iron and copper (Gross et al., 2000).

Zinc can be found in most meats, fiber sources, and dicalcium phosphate. Zinc supplements used most often include zinc oxide, zinc sulfate, zinc chloride, and zinc carbonate (Gross et al., 2000).

Copper

Copper is used by the body for iron absorption and transport and hemoglobin formation. Most of the copper found in the body is bound to the plasma protein ceruloplasmin. This protein functions as a carrier of copper and in the oxidation of plasma iron. Copper is also required for the conversion of the amino acid tyrosine to the pigment melanin and for the synthesis of connective tissues collagen and elastin, as well as for production of ATP (Case et al., 2000). Copper is needed for normal osteoblast activity during skeletal growth (Case et al., 2000).

Absorption of copper occurs throughout the intestinal tract, with the major portion being in the small intestine (Gross et al., 2000). The liver is the primary site of copper metabolism, with hepatic concentrations reflecting an animal's intake and copper status (Gross et al., 2000). Excess copper is excreted in the bile (Case et al., 2000).

Copper deficiency results in a hypochromic, microcytic anemia similar to that seen with iron deficiency. Other signs of deficiency can include depigmentation of colored hair coats and impaired skeletal development in young animals (Case et al., 2000). Excessive copper can result in interference with zinc and iron metabolism (Gross et al., 2000).

Most organ meats are rich in copper. Typical dietary supplements include cupric sulfate, cupric carbonate, and cupric chloride (Gross et al., 2000).

Selenium

Selenium is an essential component of the enzyme glutathione peroxidase, which helps to protect cellular and subcellular membranes from oxidative damage (Case et al., 2000; Gross et al., 2000). Glutathione peroxidase deactivates lipid peroxides that are formed during oxidation of cell-membrane lipids (Case et al., 2000). Vitamin E protects the polyunsaturated fatty acids (PUFAs) in cell membranes from oxidative damage, preventing the release of lipid peroxides. By reducing the number of peroxides that are formed, vitamin E spares the cellular use of selenium (Case et al., 2000). Selenium also helps to spare vitamin E by preserving the pancreas, allowing for normal fat digestion and thus normal vitamin E absorption, and by reducing the amount of vitamin E required to maintain lipid membrane integrity through the availability of glutathione peroxidase (Gross et al., 2000).

Selenium deficiencies or toxicities have not been reported in dogs and cats (Gross et al., 2000). Selenium availability in food is highly influenced by whether the selenium is from foods or is found as a supplement (Gross et al., 2000). Selenium availability averages about 20% in ingredients of animal origin and about 50% in ingredients of plant origin (Gross et al., 2000).

Sources of selenium include fish, eggs, and liver. Common supplements found in pet foods include sodium selenite and sodium selenate (Gross et al., 2000).

Iodine

Iodine is required by the body for the synthesis of the hormones thyroxine and triiodothyronine by the thyroid gland (Case et al., 2000). Thyroxine stimulates cellular oxidative processes and regulates the basal metabolic rate (Case et al., 2000). This affects thermoregulation, reproduction, growth and development, circulation, and muscle function (Gross et al., 2000).

The thyroid gland effectively traps iodine daily to ensure adequate supplies for production of the thyroid hormones (Gross et al., 2000). This trapping mechanism regulates a more or less constant iodine supply to the thyroid glands over a wide range of plasma levels (Gross et al.,

2000). Iodine requirements are influenced by physiologic state and diet (Gross et al., 2000). Lactating animals require more dietary iodine because of loss through the milk (Gross et al., 2000).

The principal sign of iodine deficiency is goiter, an enlargement of the thyroid gland (Case et al., 2000). Naturally occurring dietary deficiency does not usually occur, but diets containing "goitrogenic compounds" can lead to this. Certain compounds found in peas, peanuts, soybeans, and flaxseed can bind iodine, making it unavailable for use (Gross et al., 2000).

Fish, eggs, iodized salt, and poultry byproduct meal are good sources of iodine. Common supplements found in pet foods include calcium iodate, potassium iodide, and cuprous iodide (Gross et al., 2000).

References

Case, L.P., Carey, D.P., Hirakawa, D.A., & Daristotle, L. 2000. Vitamins and minerals. In *Canine and feline nutrition: A resource for companion animal professionals* (2nd. ed., pp. 123–128). St. Louis, MO: Mosby.

Gross, K.L., Wedekind, K.L., Cowell, C.S., Schoenherr, W.D., Jewell, D.E., Zicker, S.C., Debrakeller, J., & Frey, R.A. 2000. Nutrients. In M.S. Hand, C.D. Thatcher, R.L. Remillard, & P. Roudebush (eds.)., *Small animal clinical nutrition* (4th. ed., pp. 66–80). Marceline, MO: Walsworth Publishing for Mark Morris Institute.

Price, C.J., Bedford, P.C.G., & Sutton, J.B. 1993. Nutrients and the requirements of dogs and cats. In J.W. Simpson, R.S. Anderson, & P.J. Markwell (eds.)., *Clinical nutrition of the dog and cat* (pp. 27–30). Cambridge, MA: Blackwell Science.

8

Digestion and Absorption

The role of digestion is to break up the large complex molecules found in many nutrients into their simplest, most soluble forms so that absorption and use by the body can take place (Case et. al, 2000). The two basic types of action involved in this process are mechanical digestion, as seen with chewing and peristaltic action in the stomach and intestines, and chemical or enzymatic digestion, as seen with the splitting of chemical bonds of the complex nutrients (Case et al., 2000).

The three major types of foods requiring digestion are fats, carbohydrates, and proteins. Before fats can be absorbed, they need to be hydrolyzed to glycerol, free fatty acids, and some monoglycerides and diglycerides. Complex carbohydrates are broken down to the simple sugars of glucose, fructose, and galactose for use by the body. Proteins are hydrolyzed to their simple amino acid units and some dipeptides (Case, 2003; Case et al., 2000). The process of digestion begins when food first enters the mouth and continues until the excretion of waste products and the undigested portion of the foods in the feces (Case et al., 2000).

Digestive Tract

The digestive tract can be described as a hollow tube that starts at the mouth and continues all the way to the anus (Price et al., 1993). Within this tube, various changes take place to allow ingested nutrients to be processed and utilized (Price et al., 1993).

In all species, the mouth functions to bring food into the body and to start the initial breaking down of the food by chewing and mixing the food with saliva (Case et al., 2000). Saliva is produced in response to the sight and smell of food. It acts as a lubricant to make both chewing and swallowing easier and serves to liquefy the parts of the food that stimulate the taste buds and impart flavor to the food (Case, 2003; Case et al., 2000). Unlike many herbivores that thoroughly chew their food, dogs and cats often swallow large bites of food with little or no chewing (Case, 2003; Case et al., 2000; Price et al., 1993). The teeth of dogs and cats have few flat chewing surfaces as would be seen with an herbivore. An additional distinction can be seen with cats, which have fewer pre-molars and molars than do dogs. The additional teeth provide dogs with an increased capacity to chew and crush their food (Case, 2003; Case et al., 2000). The dental pattern seen with dogs is suggestive of a more omnivorous diet, whereas that of cats is most typical of the pattern seen with most other obligate carnivores (Case et al., 2000). Cats also lack salivary amylase, which in other animals starts carbohydrate digestion in the mouth (Kirk et al., 2000).

From the mouth, the food passes into the esophagus. When empty, the esophagus is a collapsed tube with longitudinal folds (Price et al., 1993). The lining of the esophagus contains many goblet cells that secrete a large amount of mucus to further assist in the lubrication of food during swallowing (Case et al., 2000; Price et al., 1993). At the end of the esophagus is the cardia, a muscular ring that allows food to pass into the stomach but constricts back down to prevent reflux of stomach contents into the lower esophagus (Case, 2003; Case et al., 2000; Price et al., 1993).

Swallowing involves a series of three steps; the first is under volun-tary control, and the remaining two are involuntary (Price et al., 1993). Swallowing is initiated by the formation of a bolus of food within the mouth; this is then pushed against the hard palate by the tongue and projected back into the pharynx (Price et al., 1993). Sensory receptors in the pharynx start the second step of swallowing by detecting the food bolus and closing the nasopharynx through upward movement of the soft palate. The pharyngeal muscles contract, forcing the bolus of food into the esophagus. The last phase of swallowing involves detection of the food bolus within the cranial esophagus. This detection produces a peristaltic wave, moving the food bolus down the esophagus into the stomach. A second peristaltic wave will often follow, ensuring that the food has been completely emptied into the stomach (Price et al., 1993).

The stomach acts as a reservoir for ingested food and initiates the digestion process (Price et al., 1993). By acting as a reservoir, the stomach allows for ingestion of a few large meals throughout the day rather than multiple smaller meals (Case et al., 2000). The stomach in cats is smaller than that found in dogs. Cats consume several smaller meals throughout the day (usually 10 to 20 meals), so they do not need a large-capacity stomach (Case 2003; Kirk et al., 2000).

Chemical digestion of protein starts in the stomach, as well as mixing of the food with the gastric secretions. The stomach also controls entry of food into the small intestine (Case et al., 2000). The gastric secretions are composed of mucus to protect the stomach lining and further lubricate the food, hydrochloric acid to provide the proper pH for the necessary enzymatic reactions to occur, and pepsinogen, a proteolytic enzyme (Case et al., 2000). Hydrochloric acid converts the pepsinogen into the active enzyme pepsin. This initiates the hydrolysis of protein molecules to smaller polypeptide units (Case et al., 2000).

The sight, smell, and taste of food, together with the presence of food in the stomach, stimulate the secretion of hydrochloric acid and pepsinogen.

The stomach has a built-in pacemaker that produces five slow waves per minute, some of which initiate muscular contractions (Price et al., 1993). These peristaltic movements slowly mix the ingested food with the gastric secretions, preparing it for entry into the small intestine (Case et al., 2000). Thorough mixing of the ingested food results in the production of a semifluid mass of food called chyme. Chyme must pass though the pyloric sphincter to enter the small intestine for further digestion. The pyloric sphincter acts to control the rate of passage of chyme into the small intestine. The rate of emptying can be affected by osmotic pressure, particle size, and viscosity of the chyme (Case et al., 2000). In general, larger meals have a slower rate of emptying than do small meals, liquids leave the stomach faster than do solids, and very high fat meals may cause a decrease in stomach emptying rate. Diets that contain soluble fiber can cause a decreased rate of emptying compared with diets that contain insoluble dietary fiber (Case et al., 2000). At this stage of digestion, even though the food is now semisolid chyme, the carbohydrates and fats are almost unchanged in composition, but the proteins have been partially hydrolyzed into smaller polypeptide units (Case, 2003). The majority of digestion up to this point has been primarily mechanical in nature, which is all about to change (Case et al., 2000).

The small intestine starts at the pylorus and ends at the ileocecocolic junction. It is divided into three parts, the duodenum, jejunum, and ileum. The duodenum is the first and shortest portion of the small intestine and is the site where the pancreatic and bile ducts enter the intestine (Price et al., 1993). The jejunum and ileum form the main portion of the small intestine; there is not a clear division between the different parts of the small intestine (Price et al., 1993).

Further mechanical digestion can also occur in the small intestine through the contraction of the muscle layers (Case et al., 2000). These contractions continue to mix the food with intestinal secretions, increasing the exposure of digested food particles to the surface of the intestine and slowly propelling the food mass through the intestinal tract (Case et al., 2000).

Both the pancreas and glands located in the duodenal mucosa secrete enzymes into the intestinal lumen that begin the chemical digestion of fat, carbohydrate, and protein. These enzymes include intestinal lipase, amino peptidase, dipeptidase, nucleotidase, nucleosidase, and enterokinase (Case et al., 2000). Intestinal lipase converts fat to monoglycerides, diglycerides, glycerol, and free fatty acids. Amino peptidase breaks the peptide bond located at the terminal end of the protein molecule, slowly releasing single amino acid units from the protein chain (Case et al., 2000). Dipeptidase breaks the peptide of dipeptides to release two single amino acid units. Both nucleotidase and nucleosidase hydrolyze nucleoproteins to their constituent bases and pentose sugars (Case et al., 2000). Enterokinase converts inactive trypsinogen secreted by the pancreas into its active form of trypsin; once activated, trypsin is able to activate more of itself, as well as the other protease enzymes (Price et al., 1993). The cells of the brush border that line the intestines complete the final digestion of carbohydrates through the secretion of the enzymes maltase, lactase, and sucrase. These convert the disaccharides maltose, lactose, and sucrose into the base monosaccharides of glucose, fructose, and galactose (Case et al., 2000).

The pancreas is responsible for secreting the enzymes trypsin, chymotrypsin, carypeptidase, and nuclease (Case et al., 2000). Most of these are secreted in the inactive form and are activated by other components in the small intestine after release (Case et al., 2000). The pancreas also produces lipase and amylase, which are responsible for hydrolysis of fats and starches into smaller units. The acidic chyme produced in the stomach is neutralized by bicarbonate salts produced in the pancreas; this helps to adjust the intestinal pH to provide an optimal environment for the digestive enzymes to work (Case et al., 2000).

Bile Salts

Bile salts are essential for the production of a lipid–water interface to permit lipase digestion of the triglycerides (Price et al., 1993). These are produced in the liver and stored in the gallbladder. The primary functions of bile in the small intestine are the emulsification of dietary fat and the activation of certain lipases (Case et al., 2000). The intestinal contractions ensure thorough mixing of the fat, lipase, and bile salts. This produces an emulsion of small fat droplets called micelles (Price et al., 1993).

Hormones in Digestion

Hormonal control of digestion in the small intestine involves several parts. Secretin is produced by the duodenal mucosa in response to the entry of chyme from the stomach (Case et al., 2000). Secretin stimulates the release of bicarbonate from the pancreas and controls the rate of bile release from the gall bladder. Cholecystokinin is also released from this portion of the duodenal mucosa in response to the presence of fat in the chyme. This hormone stimulates the contraction of the gallbladder, causing the release of bile into the intestinal lumen (Case et al., 2000). Cholecystokinin is also called pancreozymin, and it stimulates the release of the pancreatic enzymes (Case et al., 2000).

In dogs and cats, the chemical digestion of food is completed in the small intestine. Absorption involves the transfer by the body of digested nutrients from the intestinal lumen into the blood or lymphatic system for delivery to tissues throughout the body (Case et al., 2000). Like digestion, the primary site of absorption also occurs in the small intestine (Case et al., 2000)

Digestion after the Intestines

Amino acids units are absorbed into the enterocytes lining the small intestine by specific carriers using an energy-dependent active process. Different carriers are used for different classes of amino acids (Price et al., 1993). Once absorbed, the amino acids are sent to the liver by way of the portal vein (Price et al., 1993).

After the brush border enzymes have broken down the carbohydrates into their smallest particles, they are absorbed by the enterocytes using specific carriers in an active energy-requiring process. When the monosaccharides are in the enterocytes, they are rapidly released into the capillaries and transported to the liver (Price et al., 1993).

The micelles produced in the intestines are absorbed through a passive process into the enterocytes along with absorption of the fat-soluble vitamins (Price et al., 1993). Within the enterocyte, the fatty acids reform into triglyceride and attach to lipoproteins to form chylomicrons.

These chylomicrons are released into the lacteal, the part of the intestinal lymphatics that absorbs fats, for transportation to the liver and other tissues (Price et al., 1993). The bile remains within the intestinal lumen and eventually travels down the intestinal tract to be reabsorbed and circulated back to the liver for reuse (Case et al., 2000).

Water and electrolytes both flow across the intestinal mucosa in response to osmotic pressure (Case et al., 2000). Most of the minerals are absorbed by the body in the ionized form, meaning they carry an electrical charge. The water-soluble vitamins are absorbed via passive diffusion, although some may be absorbed by active processes when dietary levels are especially low (Case et al., 2000).

The liver further processes the absorbed monosaccharides and amino acids that arrive through the portal vein (Case et al., 2000). Some of the monosaccharides are converted to glycogen for storage, and some is secreted directly into the circulation. Some amino acids are released directly into the bloodstream, where they are available to the tissues for absorption into the cells. Excess amino acids are either converted to other nonessential amino acids or metabolized by the liver for energy (Case et al., 2000).

Large Intestine Digestion

The large intestine begins at the ileocecocolic valve and continues as the cecum, ascending, transverse and descending colon, rectum, and anus (Price et al., 1993). These divisions are clearly demarcated based on their location within the abdomen (Price et al., 1993).

The contents of the small intestine enter the colon through the ileocecocolic valve (Case et al., 2000; Price et al., 1993). The cecum is small in dogs and cats; it consists of an intestinal pocket next to the junction of the colon and small intestine and serves no known function in these animals (Price et al., 1993). In nonruminant herbivores, the cecum is quite large and has highly enhanced digestive capacities (Case et al., 2000).

The colon has three primary functions: the absorption of water and electrolytes, the fermentation of food residues by the resident bacterial population, and the storage of feces in the rectum (Price et al., 1993).

Unlike the small intestine, the large intestine has no villi and therefore has limited capacity for absorption of nutrients. It can absorb water and electrolytes quite well, although it has no mechanisms for active transport (Case et al., 2000). The absorption of water by the large intestine is very important in ensuring passage of formed feces and preventing dehydration (Price et al., 1993). Normally, water is passively absorbed from the colon following the active energy-dependent absorption of sodium chloride.

The bacterial colonies of the large intestine are able to digest some of the insoluble fiber and other nutrients in the diet that have escaped digestion in the small intestine. These bacteria are able to produce certain short-chain fatty acids (SCFAs), the most important being butyrate, which is used by the colonocytes for energy (Case et al., 2000).

Other products produced by the bacteria include various gases. When amino acids reach the colon undigested, the bacteria produce the amines indole and skatole. In addition, hydrogen sulfide gas is produced from the sulfur-containing amino acids (Case et al., 2000). Hydrogen sulfide gas, indole, and skatole impart strong odors to the feces and are responsible for flatulence (Case et al., 2000). Certain types of carbohydrates found in legumes such as soybeans are resistant to digestion by the enzymes of the small intestine. When these carbohydrates reach the colon and the resident bacteria, there is a resultant production of intestinal gas (flatulence). The degree to which flatulence and strong fecal odors occur in dogs and cats that are fed poorly digestible materials varies with the amounts and types of materials fed, as well as the resident bacteria that are present in the individual animals (Case, 2003; Case et al., 2000).

References

Case, L.P. 2003. The cat as an obligate carnivore. In *The cat: Its behavior, nutrition and health* (pp. 295–297). Ames, IA: Iowa State Press.

Case, L.P., Carey, D.P., Hirakawa, D.A., & Daristotle, L. 2000. Digestion and absorption. In *Canine and feline nutrition: A resource for companion animal professionals* (2nd. ed., pp. 53–60). St. Louis, MO: Mosby.

Kirk, C.A., Debraekeller, J., & Armstrong, P.J. 2000. Normal cats. In M.S. Hand, C.D. Thatcher, R.L. Remillard, & P. Roudebush (eds.), *Small animal clinical nutrition* (4th. ed., pp. 291–337). Marceline, MO: Walsworth Publishing for Mark Morris Institute.

Price, C.J., Bedford, P.C.G., & Sutton, J.B. 1993. Anatomy and physiology of the digestive tract. In J.W. Simpson, R.S. Anderson, & P.J. Markwell (eds.), *Clinical nutrition of the dog and cat* (pp. 1–18). Cambridge, MA: Blackwell Science.

9

Energy Balance

Energy in food is different from nutrients in that intake must be kept close to requirements. Energy balance is when an animal's intake is sufficient to meet its needs and minimal changes in the energy stored by the body occur (Case et al., 2000; Wills, 1996). Positive energy balance occurs when caloric intake exceeds energy expenditure (Case et al., 2000). In growing and pregnant animals, excess energy is converted primarily to lean body tissue; in adult animals, excess energy is stored primarily as fat with only some increase in lean tissue (Case et al., 2000; Wills, 1996). A negative energy balance occurs when caloric intake is insufficient to meet energy expenditures. Weight loss and decreases in both fat and lean body stores occur (Case et al., 2000; Wills, 1996).

Daily Energy Requirements

The daily energy requirement (DER) for dogs and cats depends on the amount of energy that the body expends on a daily basis (Case et al., 2000). Energy balance, though, is achieved by matching input and output over a long period of time (Wills, 1996). Even a small imbalance maintained over a long period of time can cause weight gain or weight loss dependent on the direction of the imbalance (Wills, 1996).

The principal mechanism for control of energy balance is thought to be through regulation of intake, although some variation in output can be important (Wills, 1996). The energy requirement of the animal and the energy density of the food will determine the quantity of food eaten on a daily basis (Wills, 1996), but a highly palatable food can lead to excess intake over energy expenditure and a poorly palatable food can lead to an insufficient intake to meet energy requirements. Regulation of intake is considered to be a negative feedback system, meaning that as weight increases, intake will decrease, and when weight decreases, intake will increase.

Energy expenditure can be divided into three major areas: resting energy requirement (RER), voluntary muscular activity, and meal-induced thermogenesis (Case et al., 2000).

Resting Energy Requirements

RER, also called resting metabolic rate, accounts for the largest portion of an animal's energy expenditure, about 60% to 75% of the total daily intake (Case et al., 2000). RER is the amount of energy used while resting quietly in a thermoneutral environment in a nonfasted animal (Case et al., 2000; Gross et al., 2000; Wills, 1996). This represents the energy required to maintain homeostasis in all of the integrated systems of the body during rest (Case et al., 2000). Factors influencing RER include gender and reproductive status, thyroid gland and autonomic nervous system function, body composition, body surface area, and nutritional status (Case et al., 2000). As an animal's lean body mass increases, or body surface area increases, RER also increases (Case et al., 2000).

Common Measurements of Energy

Basal energy requirement (BER)   The energy requirement for a normal animal in a thermoneutral environment, awake but resting in a fasting state. Also known as basal metabolic rate (BMR) or basal energy expenditure (BEE).

Resting energy requirement (RER)   The energy requirement for a normal animal at rest in a thermoneutral environment, awake but not fasted. Accounts for energy used for digestion, absorption, and metabolism of nutrients and recovery from physical activity. Also known as resting metabolic rate (RMR) or resting energy expenditure (REE).

Maintenance energy requirement (MER)   The energy requirement for a moderately active adult animal in a thermoneutral environment. Accounts for energy used for obtaining, digesting, and absorbing nutrients in an amount to maintain body weight, as well as energy used for spontaneous activity. Also known as metabolic energy expenditure (MEE).

Daily energy requirement (DER)   The energy required for average daily activity of any animal, dependent on lifestyle and activity. Includes energy necessary for work, gestation, lactation, and growth, as well as energy needed to maintain normal body temperature.

Gross energy (GE)   The total amount of heat produced by burning a food in a bomb calorimeter.

Digestible energy (DE)   The energy in a food that is remaining after accounting for losses from feces is subtracted from GE.

Metabolizable energy (ME)   The energy in a food available to the animal after losses from feces, urine, and combustible gasses are subtracted from GE.

Kilocalorie (kcal)   The energy needed to raise the temperature of 1 gram of water from 14.5°C to 15.5°C; 1 kcal = 1,000 calories.

3,500 kcal   The amount of energy required to lose or gain 1 pound (Burger, 1993; Gross et al., 2000).

Energy Expenditure

Voluntary muscular activity, or exercise, is the most variable area of energy expenditure. Muscular activity uses about 30% of the total energy expenditures (Case et al., 2000). The amount of energy expended is directly affected by the duration and intensity of the activity, although the amount of energy used can also increase as weight increases (Case et al., 2000).

Meal-induced thermogenesis is the heat produced following the intake of a meal (Case et al., 2000). The ingestion of nutrients causes heat production through the process of digestion and absorption (Case et al., 2000). The use of enzymes by the body allows these chemical reactions to occur at the relatively low temperatures found within the body. To achieve the same results in an industrial process would require much more extreme conditions of temperature, pH, or highly reactive ingredients (Burger, 1993). When a meal containing a mixture of carbohydrates, fats, and proteins is consumed, thermogenesis uses about 10% of the ingested calories to digest, absorb, metabolize, and store these nutrients (Case et al., 2000). The final amount of calories used is ultimately dependent on the composition of the diet, as well as the nutritional status of the animal (Case et al., 2000).

Adaptive thermogenesis is the change in the RER secondary to environmental stresses. These stresses include changes in ambient temperature, both heat and cold; alterations in food intake; and emotional stress (Case et al., 2000). This process allows the body to maintain the energy balance despite changes in caloric intake by being less efficient in energy use (Case et al., 2000). This process has been documented in laboratory animals and humans but has not yet been documented in companion animals (Case et al., 2000).

RER can be affected by body composition, age, caloric intake, and hormonal status (Case et al., 2000). RER also naturally decreases as an animal ages and loses lean body tissue (Case et al., 2000). Changes in RER can also occur secondary to energy restriction. When caloric intake is decreased, hormones will cause an initial decrease in requirement to conserve body tissue (Case et al., 2000; Burger, 1993). If caloric restriction continues, RER will be readjusted and will not be corrected until levels of lean body tissue return to normal (Case et al., 2000). Persistent overeating can lead to an increase in energy expenditure, in part due to the increase in lean body mass with weight gain but also due to increased meal-induced thermogenesis (Burger, 1993; Case et al., 2000).

Reproductive status affects energy requirements, with neutered animals having significantly lower estimated RER than intact animals. This is due to both a change in body composition (less lean body tissue) and a decrease in activity levels (Case et al., 2000). Intact animals tend to be more active during breeding season but also in territorial disputes that are usually not as great of a concern for a neutered animal.

Voluntary Oral Intake

Voluntary food intake is regulated by both internal physiologic controls and external cues (Case et al., 2000). The animal also receives cues from the body in the form of physical signs such as stomach contractions when empty, stimulating eating, or stomach distention when full, inhibiting eating (Burger, 1993). In addition, there are numerous neural and hormonal mechanisms that provide direct stimulation or inhibition to eating (Burger, 1993). Glucagon and insulin are examples of two hormones (Burger, 1993). Glucagon is a peptide produced in the intestines that causes a decrease in food intake. Insulin, on the other hand, is produced by the pancreas and stimulates hunger and increased food intake (Case et al., 2000). The administration of exogenous steroids can have the same effect on hunger and food intake.

External controls of food intake include stimuli such as diet palatability, food composition, and food texture and the timing and environment of meals (Case et al., 2000). Feeding a highly palatable diet is considered a primary environmental factor contributing to the overconsumption of food, which in turn leads to obesity (Case et al., 2000). This can be seen with high-fat diets, calorically dense diets, and foods that offer a variety of palatable flavors (Case et al., 2000).

Both dogs and cats have definite taste and texture preferences. The majority of dogs prefer canned and semimoist foods over dry food, with beef being the preferred flavor and cooked meat preferred over raw (Case et al., 2000). Dogs also have a strong preference for sucrose, while cats have been shown to lack the taste receptors in their tongues to even detect sugars (Case et al., 2000; Crane et al., 2000). Dogs and cats can detect several specific amino acids that are only weakly bitter to people. These amino acids and peptides help to give foods their meaty and savory aromas. They also respond to selected nucleotides and fatty acids that appear to increase the meaty taste perception in foods. A nucleotide that accumulates in decomposing meat is distasteful to cats but not to dogs. This may help explain dogs' fascination with dead animals (Crane et al., 2000). Both animals prefer warm food to cold food, with increasing palatability seen with increased fat levels in the diet (Case et al., 2000).

The timing of meals and the environment in which they are offered can affect eating behavior (Case et al., 2000). Dogs and cats rapidly become conditioned to receiving their meals at a specific time of day; this can be seen with both behavioral and physical signs (Case et al., 2000). Activity will generally increase at anticipated mealtimes, and gastric secretions and motility increase in anticipation of eating (Case et al., 2000). The number of animals being fed can also increase the amount of food consumed with each meal in dogs; this is a phenomenon called social facilitation. This causes a moderate increase in interest in food and an increased rate of eating. The degree to which this affects individual dogs can vary greatly (Case et al., 2000). Social hierarchies between dogs can also affect the amount of food eaten, with subordinate dogs eating less in the presence of dominant dogs during mealtimes (Case et al., 2000).

The frequency of meals can affect both food intake and metabolic efficiency. With increased meal frequency, there is actually an increase in energy loss through increased thermogenesis. With smaller, more frequent meals, the body uses more energy to digest, absorb, and metabolize the food than when one or two larger meals are fed (Case et al., 2000).

Nutrient Composition

The nutrient composition of the food can affect both the nutrient metabolism and the amount of food voluntarily eaten by the animal (Case et al., 2000). Most animals will decrease their intake of a high-fat diet to compensate for energy needs, although the greater caloric density of the diet with increased palatability can still cause increased energy intake in some animals (Case et al., 2000). The body is also metabolically more efficient at converting dietary fat to body fat for storage than it is at converting dietary carbohydrate or protein to body fat. Because of this, if an animal is eating calories in excess of its requirements of a high-fat diet, it will gain more weight than if it were consuming the same number of calories in a high-protein or high-carbohydrate diet (Case et al., 2000).

The addition of treats and table scraps to the diet can also override the satiety cues the body gives. These treats tend to be highly desirable and appealing, and even if full, animals will not turn them down (Case et al., 2000). This leads to an increase in energy intake and obesity because owners seldom decrease the amount of "regular food" offered to the pet. Feeding a variety of new food types can cause the same affect (Case et al., 2000).

Estimated Energy Requirements

Many formulas have been used to calculate the estimated energy requirements for animals (Table 9.1). Dogs present a unique challenge in that their sizes have one of the widest ranges in the animal kingdom, from the 4 lb. Chihuahua to the 200 lb. Great Dane. Cats tend to have a smaller range of sizes, usually between 4 and 20 lb. Some of these use

TABLE 9.1 **Formulas for calculating MER in adult maintenance in kcal/day, using body weight (BW) in kilograms.**

Canine	Feline
Inactive[1]: $99 \times BW^{0.67}$	Inactive[2,4]: $60 \times BW$
Active[1]: $132 \times BW^{0.67}$	Moderately active[4]: $70 \times BW$
Very active[1]: $160 \times BW^{0.67}$	Highly active[4]: $80 \times BW$
Endurance/performance [5]: $300 \times BW^{0.67}$	Kitten 0–3 months[4]: $250 \times BW$
<2 kg[6]: [BER $70 \times BW^{0.75}$] $\times$ 1.3–2.0	Kitten 3–5 months[4]: $130 \times BW$
>2 kg[6]: [BER $(30 \times BW) + 70$] $\times$ 1.3–2.0	<2 kg[6]: [BER $70 \times BW^{0.75}$] $\times$ 1.3–2.0
1500[3] $\times$ BSA	>2 kg[6]: [BER $(30 \times BW) + 70$] $\times$ 1.3–2.0

[1]Case et al., 2000.
[2]Donoghue, 1996.
[3]Hand et al., 2000.
[4]Case, 2003.
[5]Case, 1999.
[6]Simpson, Anderson, & Markwell, 1995.

allometric formulas, some use linear equations, and still some use body surface area (BSA). All of these formulas are helpful, but all still are only estimates of actual caloric needs. Numerous charts have also been devised that allow quick access to estimate energy needs.

Obviously, if you're using a calculator that does not have an exponential key, you'll have to use one of the linear formulas. All of these formulas have been compared, and when calculated out the results are within a reasonable distance of each other. You can also use charts that have the MER calculated out and work from these numbers. Ultimately, all energy estimates will need to be adjusted based on the desired response from the animal—weight gain, weight maintenance, or weight loss. Variability between individual animals and environmental living conditions can result in a difference ±25% of the calculated energy need (Case et al., 2000).

Using these equations and the energy density of the food, the amount of food to be fed to the individual animal can be calculated (Case et al., 2000):

Example: 10 lb. cat = 4.5 kg
MER = [(30 × 4.5 kg) + 70] × 1.3
MER = 136.36 × 1.3
MER = 177.27 kcal/day

Diet A = 326 kcal/cup
Feeding amount = 177.27/326
Feeding amount = 0.54 cup/day
This is based on a standard 8 oz. measuring cup.

TABLE 9.2 **Energy requirement for life stages.**

Life stage	Energy requirement
Canine	
Postweaning	2 × adult MER
40% Adult weight	1.6 × adult MER
80% Adult weight	1.2 × adult MER
Late gestation	1.25–1.5 × adult MER
Lactation	3 × adult MER
Prolonged physical work	2–4 × adult MER
Decreased environmental temperature	1.2–1.8 × adult MER
Feline	
Postweaning	250 kcal/kg BW
20 Weeks	130 kcal/kg BW
Late gestation	1.25 × adult MER
Lactation	3–4 × adult MER

From Gross, K.L., Wedekind, K.L., Cowell, C.S., et al. 2000. Nutrients. In M.S. Hand, C.D. Thatcher, R.L. Remillard, & P. Roudebush (eds.), *Small animal clinical nutrition* (4th. ed., pp. 31-33). Marceline, MO: Walsworth Publishing for Mark Morris Institute.

Certain life stages can result in increased energy needs (Table 9.2). These include growth, gestation, lactation, periods of strenuous physical work, and exposure to extreme environmental conditions (Case et al., 2000).

Water requirements can be expressed in one of two ways, either two to three times the dry matter intake of food, expressed in grams, or by using the MER kcal/day estimates to calculate water requirements (Case et al., 2000). The best recommendation is to have plenty of clean, fresh water available at all times, regardless of the animal's physiologic state, caloric intake, or dry matter intake (Case et al., 2000).

References

Burger, I.H. 1993. A basic guide to nutrient requirements. In I.H. Burger (ed.), *The Waltham book of companion animal nutrition* (pp. 6–10). Oxford: Butterworth-Heinemann.

Case, L.P. 1999. Nutrient requirements. In L.P. Case (ed.), *The dog: Its behavior, nutrition and health* (p. 279). Ames, IA: Iowa State Press.

Case, L.P. 2003. The cat as an obligate carnivore. In *The cat: Its behavior, nutrition and health* (pp. 295–297). Ames, IA: Iowa State Press.

Case, L.P., Carey, D.P., Hirakawa, D.A., & Daristotle, L. 2000. Energy balance. In *Canine and feline nutrition: A resource for companion animal professionals* (2nd. ed., pp. 75-88). St. Louis, MO: Mosby.

Crane, S.W., Griffin, R.W., & Messent, P.R. 2000. Introduction to commercial pet foods. In M.S. Hand, C.D. Thatcher, R.L. Remillard, & P. Roudebush (eds.), *Small animal clinical nutrition* (4th. ed., p. 123). Marceline, MO: Walsworth Publishing for Mark Morris Institute.

Donoghue, S. 1996. The underweight patient. In N.C. Kelly & J.M. Wills (eds.), *Manual of companion animal nutrition and feeding* (p. 103). Ames, IA: Iowa State Press.

Gross, K.L., Wedekind, K.L., Cowell, C.S., Schoenherr, W.D., Jewell, D.E., Zicker, S.C., Debrakeller, J., & Frey, R.A. 2000. Nutrients. In M.S. Hand, C.D. Thatcher, R.L. Remillard, & P. Roudebush (eds.), *Small animal clinical nutrition* (4th. ed., pp. 31–33). Marceline, MO: Walsworth Publishing for Mark Morris Institute.

Hand, M.S., Thatcher, C.D., Remillard, R.L., & Roudebush, P. (eds.). 2000. Appendix D. In *Small animal clinical nutrition* (4th. ed., p. 1010). Marceline, MO: Walsworth Publishing for Mark Morris Institute.

Simpson, J.W., R.S. Anderson, R.S., & Markwell, P.J. 1995. Anorexia, enteral and parenteral feeding. In *Clinical nutrition of the dog and cat* (p. 107). Cambridge, MA: Blackwell Science.

Wills, J.M. 1996. Basic principles of nutrition and feeding. In N.C. Kelly & J.M. Wills (eds.), *Manual of companion animal nutrition and feeding* (pp. 19-21). Ames, IA: Iowa State Press.

Xia, L., Weihua, L., Hong, W., et al. 2005. Pseudogenization of a sweet-receptor gene accounts for cats' indifference toward sugar. *PLoS Genetics, 1,* 27–35.

2

Nutritional Requirements of Dogs and Cats

10

History and Regulation of Pet Foods

Until the mid 1800s, dogs and cats were fed primarily table scraps with supplemental scavenging (Cowell et al., 2000). Some owners may have fed homemade food formulas made from human foods, but no commercial pet foods were available until 1860 (Case et al., 2000; Cowell et al., 2000).

The first commercial prepared dog food was produced by James Spratt, an American living in London in 1860 (Case et al., 2000; Cowell et al., 2000). On his trip across the Atlantic Ocean to England, he was unimpressed with the dry biscuits fed to his dog aboard the ship. Once in London, he developed a dry kibble, or "dog cake," that he sold to the English huntsman for their dogs (Cowell et al., 2000). Following his success with this food in England, he expanded his sales to include the United States, where production was continued until the late 1950s, when it was purchased by General Mills (Case et al., 2000; Cowell et al., 2000).

In the early 1900s, several other people saw the success that Spratt was having with his dry "dog cakes" and began to develop and sell their own formulas. In 1907, F.H. Bennett, an Englishman, developed and produced Milk-Bone dog biscuits in New York City (Case et al., 2000; Cowell et al., 2000). At that time, Milk-Bones were marketed as a complete dog food (Cowell et al., 2000).

Until the early 1920s, Spratt and Bennett were the two primary producers of commercial pet food. In the early 1920s, the Chappel brothers of Rockford, Illinois, produced the first batches of canned commercial food. They began by canning horse meat for dogs under the Ken-L-Ration brand name, following this with a dry food in the 1930s (Case et al., 2000; Cowell et al., 2000). By the mid 1920s, Samuel and Clarence Gaines of Gaines Food Company from Sherburne, New York, began selling a new type of dog food called "meal" in 100 lb. bags; this was the beginning of "Gaines Dog Meal." The food differed from previous food in that a number of dried, ground ingredients were mixed together to form the food (Case et al., 2000). The advantages of this to pet owners were that they could buy the food in fairly large quantities and very little food preparation was necessary before feeding (Case et al., 2000).

In the 1930s, the introduction of many new brands, including Cadet and Snappy, helped to make canned pet foods more popular than dry pet foods (Cowell et al., 2000). This continued until World War II, when, because pet foods were classified as "nonessential," the tin used to produce the cans was diverted to the war effort. By 1946, dry foods made up about 85% of the total pet food market in the United States (Cowell et al., 2000).

Marketing of Pet Foods

In the early years for commercial pet foods, primary marketing was through feedstores. The National Biscuit Company (Nabisco) purchased Milk-Bones in 1931 and began the first attempt to market its product in grocery stores (Case et al., 2000). At this time, selling pet foods in human food markets met with much resistance. Because most pet foods were made from byproducts of human foods, customers and store owners considered it unsanitary to sell such products next to foods that were meant for human consumption (Case et al., 2000). The convenience and economy of buying pet foods at the grocery store rapidly overcame consumer concerns (Case et al., 2000). Improved distribution and availability resulted in increased sales and popularity of commercial pet foods.

Production of Pet Foods

The development of the extrusion process of food production was introduced by researchers at the Purina Laboratories in the 1950s. Extrusion involves first mixing all of the food ingredients together and then rapidly cooking the mixtures and forcing it through an extruder. The extruder is a specialized pressure cooker that allows the food to be rapidly cooked and then shaped into bite-sized pieces. This process also increased the digestibility and palatability of the food produced (Case et al., 2000). After extrusion and drying, a coating of fat or some other palatability enhancer was usually sprayed onto the outside of the food pieces (Case et al., 2000). In 1957, Purina Dog Chow was first introduced to the commercial market. Within a year, it became the best-selling dog food in the United States and continues to maintain a number 2 position in total dog food sales today (Case et al., 2000; Cowell et al., 2000).

During this same time, General Foods created Gaines Burger, a new food that combined the convenience of dry food with the palatability of canned food. This was the first semimoist dog food product. Ralston-Purina followed this in the 1970s with the introduction of Tender Vittles, the first semimoist cat food (Cowell et al., 2000).

Science Diet, produced by Hill's Pet Nutrition, was originally produced as a consistent high-quality food for research kennels. This became the first specialty product line designed for different life stages in 1968 (Cowell et al., 2000). Hill's Pet Nutrition had been producing pet foods in cooperation with Dr. Mark Morris, Sr., since 1948—this was the Prescription Diet foods that are so familiar. The first food produced was Hill's Science Diet K/D diet canned. Originally produced in Dr. Morris' office for dogs with kidney disease in his practice, this was the first food designed to aid in the dietary management of disease (Cowell et al., 2000).

During this time, little was known about the nutrient requirements for dogs and cats. This led many manufacturers to produce the same product for both species, with only the labeling being different (Case et al., 2000). As more knowledge was acquired about different nutrient needs for dogs and cats, separate foods were formulated for each (Case et al., 2000). As knowledge continues to grow, more companies are developing diets that are specifically designed for specific life stages, physiologic states (low activity, moderate activity, and performance diets), and health problems (Case et al., 2000).

Regulatory Agencies

A number of agencies and organizations regulate the production, marketing, and sales of commercial pet foods in the United States (Case et al., 2000). The Association of American Feed Control Officials (AAFCO) was formed in 1909 and is composed of feed control officials from states and territories within the United States and Canada (Roudebush et al., 2000). AAFCO provides a forum for local, state, and federal regulatory officials to discuss and develop uniform and equitable laws, regulations, and policies regarding pet foods. AAFCO formed a permanent Pet Food Committee to address the need for information about pet nutrition and pet food regulations (Roudebush et al., 2000). The AAFCO remains the recognized information source for pet food labeling, ingredient definition, official terms, and standardized feed testing methodology (Roudebush et al., 2000). Because the AAFCO is an association and not an official regulatory body, its policies must be voluntarily accepted by state feed control officials for actual implementation (Case et al., 2000). Pet food regulations can vary from state to state, and use of the AAFCO's policy statements and regulations promotes uniformity in feed regulations throughout the United States (Case et al., 2000). Today, AAFCO ensures that nationally marketed pet foods are uniformly labeled and nutritionally adequate (Case et al., 2000).

During the 1990s, AAFCO developed the practical Nutrient Profiles to be used as standards for the formulation of dog and cat foods. The profiles are based on ingredients commonly include in commercial foods, and nutrient levels are expressed for processed foods at the time of feeding (Case et al., 2000). Prior to this, nutrient minimums were based on the recommendations of the National Research Council (NRC) (Roudebush et al., 2000). The NRC recommendations are based on data obtained from the use of purified foods, with the assumption of 100% nutrient availability for only one life stage, and gave only minimum levels without any safety margins (Roudebush et al., 2000). The Nutrient Profiles provide suggested levels of nutrients to be included in pet foods rather than minimum levels, as do the NRC recommendations, as well as maximum levels of selected nutrients (Case et al., 2000). AAFCO also publishes minimum feeding protocols for dog and cat foods. These minimum feeding protocols are used by pet food manufacturers to substantiate the nutritional adequacy of pet foods using feeding trials and to determine the metabolizable energy found in dog and cat food (Roudebush et al., 2000).

The U.S. Food and Drug Administration (FDA) requires that all pet food manufacturers provide proper identification of pet foods, a net quantity statement on the label, proper listing of ingredients, and the manufacturer's name and address and use acceptable manufacturing procedures (Case et al., 2000; Roudebush et al., 2000). Feed control officials within each state inspect facilities and enforce these regulations, although the FDA is authorized to take direct action if necessary to address any violations (Case et al., 2000; Roudebush et al., 2000). The Center for Veterinary Medicine (CVM), a department of the FDA, regulates the use of any health claims on pet food labels. One type of health claim, a drug claim, is defined as the assertion or implication that the consumption of a food may help in the treatment, prevention, or reduction of a particular disease or diseases (Case et al., 2000). If a health claim is considered a drug claim, the CVM will not allow its use on the label (Case et al., 2000).

The U.S. Department of Agriculture (USDA) is responsible for ensuring that pet foods are clearly labeled to prevent human consumers from mistaking these products for human foods (Case et al., 2000; Roudebush et al., 2000). The USDA inspects animal ingredients used in pet foods to ensure proper handling and to guarantee that such ingredients are not used in human foods (Case et al., 2000; Roudebush et al., 2000). The USDA is also responsible for inspection and regulation of animal research facilities. All kennels and catteries that are operated by pet food companies, private groups, or universities must fulfill USDA requirements for physical structure, record keeping, housing and care of animals, and sanitation (Case et al., 2000; Roudebush et al., 2000). Once these facilities have passed their initial certification, they are subject to unannounced inspections by the USDA at least once yearly (Case et al., 2000; Roudebush et al., 2000).

Some pet food manufacturers maintain their own kennels, while other contract their feeding trials out to private research kennels or universities. Long-term feeding trials make up a large portion of the testing conducted on quality commercial pet foods. The USDA ensures that these facilities maintains proper care of their animals and conform to recommended sanitation practices (Case et al., 2000).

The National Research Council (NRC) is a private, nonprofit organization that evaluates and compiles research conducted by others. The NRC functions as the working portion of the National Academy of Sciences, the National Academy of Engineers, and The Institute of Medicine (Roudebush et al., 2000). The NRC was created in 1916 in response to the increased need for scientific and technical services during World War I (Roudebush et al., 2000). It is not part of the U.S. government, is not an enforcement agency, and is not a basic research organization with laboratories of its own (Roudebush et al., 2000). The NRC does not regulate the pet food industry and has requested that its recommendations not be used to substantiate nutritional adequacy of pet foods (Roudebush et al., 2000).

In 1958, the Pet Food Institute (PFI) was organized to represent manufacturers of commercially prepared dog and cat food in the United States (Case et al., 2000; Roudebush et al., 2000). The PFI works closely with the Pet Food Committee of the AAFCO to evaluate current regulations and to make recommendations to changes (Case et al., 2000;

Roudebush et al., 2000). The PFI also works closely with veterinarians, humane groups, and local animal control officers to sponsor public and owner education programs that encourage responsible dog and cat ownership (Roudebush et al., 2000). They do not have any direct regulatory powers over production of pet foods, pet food testing, or statements included on labels, although they do represent the pet food industry before legislative and regulatory bodies at the federal and state levels (Roudebush et al., 2000).

Individual states are responsible for adopting and enforcing pet food regulations. Many, but not all, have adopted regulations that follow those established by AAFCO. Pet food regulation and enforcement is most states are administered by the State Department of Agriculture, Regulatory and Protection Division or State Chemist (Roudebush et al., 2000).

Most of the control over the nutrient content of pet foods, ingredient nomenclature, and label claims is regulated by AAFCO. The Model Feed Bill that the AAFCO developed and implemented is a template for state legislation (Case et al., 2000). Each year, the AAFCO publishes an official document that includes a section containing the current regulations for pet foods. These regulations govern the definition and terms, label format, brand and product names, nutrient guarantee claims, types of ingredients, drug and food additives, statements of caloric content, and descriptive terms that are to be used with or included in commercial pet foods (Case et al., 2000). The AAFCO-sanctioned feeding protocols for proving nutritional adequacy and metabolizable energy are also included in this document (Roudebush et al., 2000).

Regulations

The definition and terms section of the AAFCO's pet food regulations identify the Principal Display Panel (PDP) as part of the container's label that is intended to be displayed to the customer for retail sales (Case et al., 2000). Statements that are allowed on labels are described and strictly regulated; these are called "statements of nutritional adequacy" or "purpose of the product." If a product states that it is "complete and balanced nutrition for all stages of life," the claim must be substantiated through one of two ways (Case et al., 2000). The first way involves the use of a series of feeding trials to demonstrate that the food satisfactorily supports the health in a group of dogs or cats throughout all life stages of gestation, lactation, and growth (Case et al., 2000). The second way requires that the manufacturer formulate the food to contain ingredients in quantities that are sufficient to provide the estimated nutrient requirements for all life stages in the dog or cat (Case et al., 2000). This can be shown through simple calculation of ingredients using standard ingredient tables or through laboratory analysis of nutrients (Case et al., 2000). The AAFCO Nutrient Profiles for dog and cat foods are used as the standard against which to measure nutrient content (Case et al., 2000). The AAFCO also requires that all products labeled "complete and balanced" include specific feeding directions on the product label (Case et al., 2000).

Brand name refers to the name by which a pet food manufacturer's products are identified and distinguished from other pet foods (Case et al., 2000). The AAFCO regulates both brand and product names (Case et al., 2000). Any product claims of "new and improved" are only allowed to be stated on the PDP and can be used for a maximum of 6 months (Case et al., 2000).

The AAFCO identifies acceptable terms for designating the guaranteed analysis for specific nutrients. Comparisons that are made between nutrient levels in the pet food and the AAFCO Nutrient Profiles must be listed in the same units as those used in the published profile (Case et al., 2000). AAFCO also requires that no pet food, with the exception of those labeled as sauces, gravies, juices, or milk replacers, contain a moisture level greater than 78% (Case et al., 2000).

Artificial food colors can be added to pet foods only if they have been shown to be harmless to pets (Case et al., 2000). Such additives are approved and listed by the FDA (Case et al., 2000).

In 1994, AAFCO accepted the inclusion of an optional caloric content statement on pet food labels (Case et al., 2000). This statement must be presented separately from the guaranteed analysis table, and the energy must be expressed in ME in units of kcal/kg. The caloric content may also be expressed as kcal/lb, cup, or other commonly used household measuring unit (Case et al., 2000). This claim must be substantiated either by calculation using modified Atwater factors or through feeding trials following AAFCO protocols (Case et al., 2000). The method used must be stated on the label (Case et al., 2000).

In 1998, the newest addition to the AAFCO regulations specifies the acceptable use of the terms "light/lite," "less or reduced calories," "lean," "low fat," and "less or reduced fat" (Case et al., 2000). Specific maximum energy contents are designated for all pet foods marketed using the term "light/lite." A food designated as "less or reduced calories" must include the percentage of reduction from the product of comparison and a caloric content statement (Case et al., 2000). The terms "lean" and "less fat" must provide the maximum percentages of fat within different categories of dog and cat food and include the percentage of reduction from the product of comparison (Case et al., 2000).

References

Case, L.P., Carey, D.P., Hirakawa, D.A., & Daristotle, L. 2000. History and regulation of pet foods. In *Canine and feline nutrition: A resource for companion animal professionals* (2nd. ed., pp. 143–151). St. Louis, MO: Mosby.

Cowell, C.S., Stout, N.P., Brinkerman, M.F., et al. 2000. Making commercial pet foods. In M.S. Hand, C.D. Thatcher, R.L. Remillard, & P. Roudebush (eds.), *Small animal clinical nutrition* (4th. ed., p. 129). Marceline, MO: Walsworth Publishing for Mark Morris Institute.

Roudebush, P., Dzanis, D.A., Debraekeleer, J., & Brown, R.G.. 2000. Pet food labels. In M.S. Hand, C.D. Thatcher, R.L. Remillard, & P. Roudebush (eds.), *Small animal clinical nutrition* (4th. ed., pp. 147–150). Marceline, MO: Walsworth Publishing for Mark Morris Institute.

11

Pet Food Labels

Pet food labels are legal documents regulated primarily by the Association of American Feed Control Officials (AAFCO). They are under the jurisdiction of the U.S. Food and Drug Administration (FDA). Regulations that apply to pet food labeling and testing of foods for nutritional adequacy are published in the AAFCO manual (Buffington et al., 2004). This manual is updated yearly and also provides definitions for the various terms used in pet food labeling (Buffington et al., 2004).

Definition of Terms

Complete   A nutritionally adequate feed for animals other than humans; by specific formula, it is compounded to be fed as a sole ration and is capable of maintaining life and/or promoting production without any additional substance being consumed except water (Buffington et al., 2004).

Balanced   A term that may be applied to a diet, ration, or feed having all the required nutrients in proper amounts and proportions based upon recommendations of recognized authorities in the field of animal nutrition, such as the National Research Council (NRC), for a given set of physiological requirements. The species for which it is intended and the functions, such as maintenance or maintenance plus reproduction, shall be specified (Buffington et al., 2004).

TABLE 11.1. **Percentage of content in a food (using chicken as an example).**

Product	Content
Chicken	Chicken must constitute at least 70% of the total product.
Chicken dinner, chicken platter, chicken entree	Chicken must constitute at least 10% of the total product.
With chicken	Chicken must constitute at least 3% of the total product.
Chicken flavor	Chicken must be recognizable by the pet, usually less than 3% of the total product.
Canned foods	Moisture must not be greater than 78%.
Gravy, stew, broth, sauce, juice, or milk replacer	Moisture can be greater than 78%.

Regulations

Current regulations require that labels for all pet foods manufactured and sold in the United States contain the following items: product name; net weight; name and address of the manufacturer; guaranteed analysis for crude protein, crude fat, crude fiber, and moisture; list of ingredients in descending order of predominance by weight; the term "dog food" or "cat food"; and a statement of nutritional adequacy or purpose of the product (Buffington et al., 2004; Case et al., 2000). A statement must also be included that indicates the method used to substantiate the nutritional adequacy claim—this can be either through the AAFCO feeding trials or by formulating the feed to meet AAFCO Nutrient Profiles. An expiration date indicating the time span from the date of production to the date of expiration of the product is optional, as is a "best if used by" date (Buffington et al., 2004; Case et al., 2000).

Principal Display Panel

The required information can be found on either the principal display panel (PDP) or the information panel. The PDP is defined by the FDA as "the part of the label that is most likely to be displayed, presented, shown or examined under customary conditions of display for retail sale" (Roudebush et al., 2000). This is the primary means of attracting the consumer's attention to a product and should immediately communicate the product identity. The information panel is defined as

TABLE 11.2. Sample label.

Dr K's Natural Food 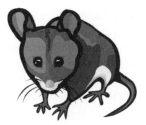 Field Mouse For Cats Complete and Balance as Nature Designed for adult maintenance	INGREDIENTS: Water sufficient for processing; Michigan-grown, whole, ground, wild field mouse. GUARANTEED ANALYSIS: Crude protein min. 20%, crude fat min. 10%, crude fiber max. 1%, moisture max. 65%, ash max. 4% AAFCO feeding studies substantiate complete and balanced for adult maintenance Manufactured by MVS, Southfield MI USA (748) 577–1156 Feeding Recommendations:

Size	1–5#	6–10#	11–15#	16–20#
Amt fed	.5–.6 can	.6–1 can	1–1.5 can	1.5–2 can

"that part of the label immediately contiguous and to the right of the PDP" and usually contains information about the product (Roudebush et al., 2000).

The product identity is the primary means of identification of pet foods by consumers (Roudebush et al., 2000). In the United States, the

TABLE 11.3. Important elements found on pet food labels in the United States and Canada.

Principal Display Panel	Information Panel

Product identity (required)
    Manufacturer's name
    Brand name
    Product name
Designator or statement of
  intent (required)
Net weight (required)
Product vignette or picture (optional)
Nutritional claim (optional)
Bursts or flags (optional)
	Ingredient statement
	  (required)
	Guaranteed analysis (required)
	Nutritional adequacy statement (required)
	Feeding guidelines (required)
	Manufacturer or distributor (required)
	Universal product code (optional)
	Batch information (optional)
	Freshness date (optional)

product identity must legally include a product name but may also include a manufacturer's name, a brand name, or both (Roudebush et al., 2000). The brand name is the name by which the pet food products of a given company are identified (Roudebush et al., 2000). The product name provides information about the individual identity of a particular product within that brand (Roudebush et al., 2000).

The PDP must identify the species for which the food is intended, such as "dog food" or "cat food." This statement is intended to help guide consumers' purchases (Buffington et al., 2004). This does not mean that the food cannot be fed to an alternate species but that it has been tested and formulated only for the indicated species. This is called the "designator" or "statement of intent" (Roudebush et al., 2000).

The net weight indicates the amount of food in the specific container, often given in pounds or grams or both (Buffington et al., 2004). This is found on the PDP and must be placed within the bottom 30% of panel (Roudebush et al., 2000).

A product vignette refers to any vignette, graphic, or pictorial representation of a product on a pet food label (Roudebush et al., 2000). The product vignette should not misrepresent the contents of the package by looking better than the actual product or ingredients (Roudebush et al., 2000).

Nutrition statements on the PDP include the terms "complete and nutritious," "100% nutritious," "100% complete nutrition," or similar designations. These claims must be substantiated by a nutritional adequacy statement on the information panel (Roudebush et al., 2000).

Bursts and flags are areas of the PDP that are designated to highlight information or provide specific information with visual impact (Roudebush et al., 2000). New products, formula or ingredient changes, and improvements in taste are most often highlighted (Roudebush et al., 2000). "New" or "new and improved" can only appear on the label for six months, while comparisons such as "preferred 5 to 1 over the leading national brand" can appear on the label for 1 year, unless it is resubstantiated (Roudebush et al., 2000).

Information Panel

The information panel is usually the second place that consumers look for information about a food they are buying (Case et al., 2000). The list of ingredients must be arranged in decreasing order by predominance by weight. The terms used to describe the products must be those assigned for that product by the AAFCO or names that are commonly accepted as a standard in the feed industry (Case et al., 2000). No single ingredient can be given undue emphasis, nor can designators of quality be included (Case et al., 2000).

Most grocery store and generic brands are formulated as "variable formula diets" (Case et al., 2000). This means that the ingredients used in the food will vary from batch to batch, depending on market availability and pricing. In contrast, most premium foods sold in feedstores, in pet stores, and through veterinarians are produced using fixed formulas (Case et al., 2000). Although the cost for a fixed formula food may be more than that for a variable formula diet, the consistency between batches of food is a distinct advantage to the dog or cat consuming the food (Case et al., 2000).

The ingredient list can give no indicator of the quality of the ingredients used in the food. These ingredients can vary in digestibility, amino acid content and availability, mineral availability, and the amount of indigestible materials they contain (Case et al., 2000). Unfortunately, there is no way to determine quality from the ingredient list. In fact, some premium foods with very high-quality ingredients may have an ingredient list that is almost identical to that of a generic food that contains poor-quality ingredients with low digestibility and poor nutrient availability (Case et al., 2000). This can be seen in products that claim to be "the same as" another higher priced product. As with most anything else, you get what you pay for.

Another misleading practice is the splitting of ingredients to place them lower on the ingredient list. This occurs when several different forms of the same product are listed separately (e.g., wheat germ meal, wheat middlings, wheat bran, wheat flour). Because the requirement is to list by weight, by splitting the ingredients, they each weigh less and can be placed farther down the ingredient list when in fact they compose a major portion of the product. Dry ingredients also appear lower on the list than those that are naturally higher in moisture. This allows most "meat" products to appear higher on the ingredient list than the dry grains and starches, which may actually be found in a higher percentage in the diet (Roudebush et al., 2000).

Pet food additives such as vitamins, minerals, antioxidant preservatives, antimicrobial preservatives, humectants, coloring agents, flavors, palatability enhancers, and emulsifying agents that are listed by the manufacturer must also be included on the ingredient list (Roudebush et al., 2000).

In the United States, pet food manufacturers are required to include minimum percentages for crude protein and crude fat and maximum percentages for crude fiber and moisture (Roudebush et al.,

TABLE 11.4. **Common pet food ingredients.**

Description	Example	Contribution to diet
Meat (muscle)	Skeletal muscle, tongue, diaphragm, heart	Animal fat, protein, energy
Meat byproducts	Lung, spleen, kidney, brain, blood, bone, intestine	Animal fat, protein, energy
Meat meal, meat and bone meal, fish meal, blood meal	Dry rendered product from animal tissue	Animal fat, protein, energy
Cereals	Corn, wheat, oats, barley, corn gluten meal	Carbohydrate, protein, fiber, energy
Soy flour, soy meal	Vegetable protein source including textured vegetable protein (TVP)	Protein, texture/chunks (usually the meaty chunks in foods)
Animal fat, vegetable oil	Tallow, chicken fat, corn oil, soy oil	Fats, fatty acids, essential fatty acids, energy
Egg	Egg powder	Protein of high biologic value
Milk	Skim milk powder, whey	Milk protein
Grain nulls, root crops	Bran, beet pulp	Dietary fiber
Humectants	Sugars, salt, glycerol	Reduction in water availability, energy
Digest	Hydrolysed liver or intestine	Flavor and palatability enhancer, some protein and fat
Preservatives	Sodium benzoate, sodium and potassium sorbate	Retard spoilage from molds and bacteria
Flavors	Natural and artificial and "nature identical" flavors; process reacted flavors; key character compounds	Improvement in taste, smell, and mouth feel
Coloring agents	Natural and artificial colorings	Improvement in owner appeal
Aromas	Natural and artificial aromas and tones	Improvement in owner and animal appeal
Vitamins, minerals	Vitamin and mineral premixes	Nutrients and dietary balance
Antioxidants	BHT, BHA, ascorbic acid, mixed tocopherols (vitamin E)	Prevents fat rancidity

From Wills, J.M. 1996. Food types and evaluation. In N.C. Kelly & J.M. Wills (eds.), *Manual of companion animal nutrition and feeding* (p. 34). Ames, IA: Iowa State Press.

2000). These percentages generally indicate the "worst case" levels for these nutrients in the food and may not accurately reflect the exact or typical amounts included (Roudebush et al., 2000). Also notice that these indicate only minimum or maximum values found in the foods. Actual values may differ dramatically.

Crude protein is the estimate of the total protein in a food that is obtained by multiplying analyzed levels of nitrogen by a constant (Case et al., 2000; Roudebush et al., 2000). Crude protein is an index of protein quantity but does not give an indication of amino acid content or protein quality or digestibility (Case et al., 2000; Roudebush et al., 2000).

Crude fat is an estimate of the lipid content of a food that is obtained through extraction of the food with ether (Case et al., 2000; Roudebush et al., 2000). This procedure also isolates certain organic acids, oils, pigments, alcohols, and fat-soluble vitamins. But it may not be able to isolate some complex lipids such as the phospholipids (Case et al., 2000; Roudebush et al., 2000).

Crude fiber represents the organic residue that remains after the plant material has been treated with dilute acid and alkali solvents and after mineral components have been extracted (Case et al., 2000; Roudebush et al., 2000). Although crude fiber is used to report the fiber content of commercial foods, it usually underestimates the true level of fiber found in the food (Roudebush et al., 2000).

The amount of water found in an individual product can significantly affect the values of the other nutrients listed on the guaranteed analysis, because most pet foods display nutrients on an "as-fed" basis rather than on a "dry-matter" basis (Case et al., 2000; Roudebush et al., 2000). An as-fed basis means that the percentages of nutrients were calculated directly, without accounting for the proportion of water in a product (Case et al., 2000; Roudebush et al., 2000). It is important to convert these guarantees to dry-matter basis when comparing foods of differing moisture contents, such as canned versus dry foods (Case et al., 2000; Roudebush et al., 2000). Most dry foods contain 6% to 10% water, whereas canned foods can contain up to 78% water (Case et al., 2000; Roudebush et al., 2000). It is also possible to use metabolizable energy when comparing different foods; this will give you the percentage of each nutrient in the food on an as-fed basis, taking into account the different caloric amounts of each nutrient in the food.

Maximum ash guarantees are not required in the United States but are often included on pet food labels (Roudebush et al., 2000). Ash consists of the noncombustible materials in food, usually composed of salt and other minerals. High ash content in dry and semimoist foods generally indicates high magnesium content (Roudebush et al., 2000). The ash content of canned cat foods usually correlates poorly with the magnesium content (Roudebush et al., 2000).

With the exception of treats or snacks, all pet foods that are in interstate commerce must contain a statement and validation of nutritional adequacy (Case et al., 2000; Roudebush et al., 2000). Current AAFCO regulations allow four primary types of nutritional adequacy statements:

Complete and balanced for all life stages   The food has been formulated to provide complete and balanced nutrition for gestation, lactation, growth, and maintenance.

Limited claim   The food provides complete and balanced nutrition for a particular life stage such as adult maintenance.

Intermittent or supplemental   The food has been formulated for only intermittent or supplemental use.

Therapeutic   The food is intended for therapeutic use under the supervision of a veterinarian (Case et al., 2000; Roudebush et al., 2000).

The foods must also indicate what method was used to establish the nutritional adequacy claims. The use of feeding trials is the most thorough and reliable method of evaluation. The terms "feeding tests," "AAFCO feeding test protocols," or "AAFCO feeding studies" all validate that the product has undergone feeding tests with dogs or cats. If the substantiation claim states only that the food has met the AAFCO's Nutrient Profiles, this indicates that feeding trials were not conducted on the food (Case et al., 2000; Roudebush et al., 2000). The nutrient levels can be calculated in a laboratory after production or the diet can merely be formulated using a standard table of ingredients (Case et al., 2000). Neither of these methods takes into account digestibility or availability of individual nutrients or loss of nutrients through processing or excesses found in the ingredients.

Feeding guidelines are required on all foods labeled as complete and balanced for any life stage (Roudebush et al., 2000). These directions must be given in common terms and must appear prominently on the label. At a minimum, these should state "feed (weight/unit of product) per (weight unit) or dog or cat" with a stated frequency. The guidelines are general at best. Because of individual variations, specific animals may require more or less food than recommended on the label to maintain optimal body condition and health (Roudebush et al., 2000).

A statement of caloric content may be included in the information panel but is not required. It must be separate from the guaranteed analysis and appear under the heading of "caloric content." The statement is usually based on kilocalories of metabolizable energy (ME) on an as-fed basis and must be expressed as kilocalories per kilograms of product. It may also be given as kilocalories per familiar household measure, such as kcal/cup or kcal/can (Roudebush et al., 2000).

In the United States, the name and address of the manufacturer, distributor, or dealer of the pet food must be found on the label, usually on the information panel (Roudebush et al., 2000). This information is not required to be complete and may only include the distributor and city of origin. Most premium foods include their name, mailing address, telephone number with hours of operations, and possibly a Website address. This makes it much easier for the consumer to contact the manufacturer with any problems or questions regarding the product.

Although not a legal requirement, most manufacturers include the Universal Product Code (UPC) or bar code on the label. Other information, such as batch numbers and date of manufacture, can also frequently be found on the labels. There may also be a freshness date included on the label (Roudebush et al., 2000).

References

Buffington, C.A., Holloway, C., & Abood, S.K. 2004. Diet and feeding factors. In *The manual of veterinary dietetics* (pp. 43–48). St. Louis, MO: Elsevier.

Case, L.P., Carey, D.P., Hirakawa, D.A., & Daristotle, L. 2000. Pet food labels. In *Canine and feline nutrition: A resource for companion animal professionals* (2nd. ed., pp. 153–163). St. Louis, MO: Mosby.

Roudebush, P., Dzanis, D.A., Debraekeleer, J., & Brown, R.G. 2000. Pet food labels. In M.S. Hand, C.D. Thatcher, R.I. Remillard, & P. Rooudebush (eds.). Small Animal clinical nutrition (4th. ed., pp. 151–157). Marceline, MO: Walsworth Publishing for Mark Morris Institute.

Wills, J.M. 1996. Food types and evaluation. In N.C. Kelly & J.M. Wills (eds.), *Manual of companion animal nutrition and feeding* (p. 34). Ames, IA: Iowa State Press.

12

Nutrient Content of Pet Foods

Nutrient content refers not only to the exact levels of the various nutrients in the food but also to the digestibility and availability of all of the essential nutrients (Case et al., 2000). There are four different ways that the nutrient content of a product can be determined (Hand et al., 2000): a laboratory analysis of the final product can be done, the target values can be obtained from the manufacturer, nutrient content can be calculated based on published values for the ingredients, and the information found on the label guaranteed analysis and typical analysis can be used (Hand et al., 2000).

Using the label guaranteed analysis is the least accurate, and is not recommended due to severe limitations and discrepancies in the calculated values (Hand et al., 2000).

Calculating nutrient content based on published values of ingredients also has limitations; there is a lack of complete and accurate data for the nutrient content of many ingredients used in commercial pet foods. Because of this, manufacturers rely on lists that contain approximations of the types of ingredients that are used (Case et al., 2000). These lists may also contain information that is outdated or misleading resulting in inaccurate values being used (Case et al., 2000). Since the quality of the ingredients is not taken into account when using the calculation method, this can affect the level and availability of nutrients in the finished product (Case et al., 2000). Processing methods can further affect ingredient quality with nutrient losses occurring during both processing and storage (Case et al., 2000). Studies have shown that digestibility and nutrient availability of animal-based and plant-based ingredients are significantly affected by processing methods (Case et al., 2000). This method would likely be used for determining the nutrient content of home made diets, though adequate time and knowledge to perform the calculations would be a major limitation (Hand et al., 2000).

Most pet food manufacturers will supply target values for the nutrient content of their foods upon request (Hand et al., 2000). Though these values often reflect actual average nutrient levels, occasionally they will vary significantly from the actual values found in the food (Hand et al., 2000). Since there are no laws governing the accuracy of target nutrient levels, the manufacturer does not have to have the food within these levels (Hand et al., 2000). Overall, these values should be a reasonable approximation of nutrient levels, and will be adequate for most instances.

The most accurate way to determine nutrient content is through laboratory analysis of the final product; this is called a proximate analysis (Case et al., 2000). A proximate analysis tests for a limited number of parameters, including moisture content, crude protein, crude fat, ash (minerals) and fiber contents (Case et al., 2000). Nitrogen-free extract (NFE) represents a rough estimation of the soluble carbohydrate content of the food and can be calculated by simple subtraction. Starting at 100%, subtract the percentages given for moisture, protein, fat, ash and fiber. What is left is the NFE (Hand et al., 2000). The guaranteed analysis panel is generated from the proximate analysis results, and reports only the maximum or minimum levels (Case et al., 2000).

Digestibility provides a measure of the final diet's quality because it directly determines the proportion of nutrients in the food that are available for absorption into the body (Case et al., 2000). Currently, AAFCO regulations do not require companies to determine digestibility of their foods (Case et al., 2000). Feeding trials is the process used to determine digestibility of nutrients (Case et al., 2000). Information about the nutrient content of a diet has little meaning if the digestibility is unknown (Case et al., 2000). If you have two diets that each contain 28% protein, if the digestibility of one diet is 70%, and the digestibility of the second diet is 85% the actual protein available to the animal is less than 20% in the first diet, and over 24% in the second diet (Case et al., 2000). So even though laboratory analysis would show that they have similar protein contents, digestibility shows that the second diet provides significantly more digestible protein than would the first diet (Case et al., 2000).

Digestibility also affects fecal volume, form and frequency. As a diets digestibility increases, fecal volume decreases significantly, additionally a highly digestible diet produces firm and well-formed feces (Case et al., 2000).

Manufacturers are not required to conduct feeding trials to determine digestibility of their foods. Reputable companies that produce quality products always conduct these trials to ensure that their foods contain levels of nutrients that will meet an animal's daily requirements for absorption into the body (Case et al., 2000).

Feeding Trials

In the United States, the AAFCO testing procedure for adult maintenance diets are done over a period of six months, require only eight animals per group and monitor only a limited number of parameters (Hand et al., 2000). Passing such tests does not ensure that long-term nutrition or health related problems will not occur, or that problems with a provenance rate less than 15% won't be seen (Hand et al., 2000). The protocols are also not designed to ensure optimal growth or maximize physical activity (Hand et al., 2000). If these factors are of concern, additional long-term feeding trials need to be evaluated. Numerous premium pet food manufactures conduct long-term studies looking at optimizing the response to various nutrients as well as therapeutic treatment protocols.

Food Comparisons

When trying to compare various foods or different types, what method is best to use? If foods are compared on a dry-matter basis (DMB), differences seen with different food types can be eliminated, but differences in energy content are not addressed. The energy content for protein and carbohydrates is about 3.5 kcal/g while fat is about 8.5 kcal/g. To accurately evaluate different diets the nutrient density should be evaluated as a proportion of metabolizable energy (ME) (Case et al., 2000). Nutrient density accounts for differences in both water content and energy content, and expresses nutrient levels in pet foods based on the energy available for the animal to use as metabolizable energy (Case et al., 2000).

Nutrient density is expressed as grams/100 kcal of ME for each nutrient (Case et al., 2000). Since all animals are fed to meet their energy requirements, the amount of food consumed and the amount of nutrients received depends on the energy density of the food (Case et al., 2000). When an animal is fed a calorically dense food, the percentage of nutrients by weight in these foods must be higher to meet the needs for all of the essential nutrients since less food will be consumed by the animal (Case et al., 2000).

The easiest way to express nutrients is as a percentage of ME or as units per 1,000 kcal of ME, instead of a percentage of weight. Nutrient densities of foods with different moisture contents can be compared because water does not contribute any calories to the distribution (Case et al., 2000). Unfortunately, this method does not take into account the calories in the foods or the amount that must be consumed by the animal to meet energy requirements (Case et al., 2000).

Caloric distribution is helpful when trying to find a diet that is higher or lower than another diet in certain nutrients. The three primary nutrients that are evaluated are protein, fat and carbohydrates. These are usually given as pie charts or line charts in the product reference guides available from the manufacturers.

The two last diets in Table 12.1 are the same brand; notice the different caloric distribution between the canned and dry foods.

If the grams of nutrients/100 gram of food is not given, than using the guaranteed analysis and kcal/100 grams the following formula can

---

TABLE 12.1. **Examples of nutrient density and caloric distribution from Eukanuba Veterinary Diets Product Reference Guide.**

DIET A: DRY FOOD (RENAL DIET)

Nutrient Density (g/1,000 kcal ME)
Crude protein: 47.21
Crude fat: 33.05
Crude fiber: 5.63
Carbohydrate: 135.84

Guaranteed Analysis
Crude protein: 18% DM
Crude Fat: 12%
Crude Fiber: 4%
Moisture: 10%

Metabolizable Calories
Protein: 18%
Fat: 31%
Carbohydrate: 51%

Caloric Distribution

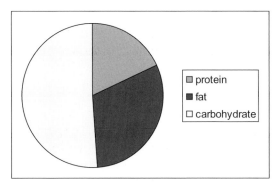

DIET B: CANNED FOOD (RECOVERY DIET)
Nutrient Density (g/1,000 kcal ME)
Crude protein: 74.80
Crude fat: 71.05
Crude fiber: 2.75
Carbohydrate: 13.20

Guaranteed Analysis
Crude protein: 14%
Crude fat: 12%
Crude fiber: 1%
Ash: 2.5%

Metabolizable Calories
Protein: 29%
Fat: 66%
Carbohydrate 5%

Caloric Distribution

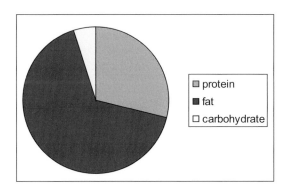

DIET: C DRY FOOD (INTESTINAL DIET)

(continued)

Table 12.1 *continued*

Nutrient density (g/1,000 kcal ME)
Crude protein: 58.85
Crude fat: 24.64
Crude fiber: 4.87
Carbohydrate: 128.96

Guaranteed Analysis
Crude protein: 22%
Crude fat: 9%
Crude fiber: 4%
Moisture: 10%

Metabolizable Calories
Protein: 24%
Fat: 24%
Carbohydrate: 52%

Caloric Distribution

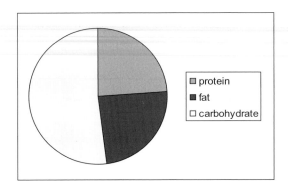

DIET: D CANNED FOOD (INTESTINAL DIET)

Nutrient Density (gm/1,000 kcal ME)
Crude protein: 78.03
Crude fat: 47.16
Crude fiber: 4.65
Carbohydrate: 69.80

Guaranteed Analysis
Crude protein: 7%
Crude fat: 2.8%
Crude fiber: 1%
Moisture: 78%

Metabolizable Calories
Protein: 30%
Fat: 44%
Carbohydrate: 26%

Caloric Distribution

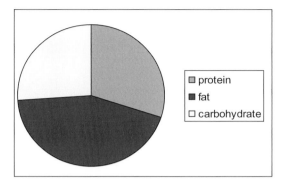

TABLE 12.2 **Nutrients as a percentage of metabolizable energy.**

Total calories in 100 g of food

Protein = 3.5 kcal/g × grams in food
Fat = 8.5 kcal/g × grams in food
Carbohydrate = 3.5 kcal/g × grams in food
Total calories/100 g = protein calories + fat calories + carbohydrate calories

Percentage of ME contributed by each nutrient (caloric distribution)

Protein = (protein calories/100 g divided by total calories/100 gram) × 100 = % ME
Fat = (fat calories/100 g divided by total calories/100 gram) × 100 = % ME
Carbohydrate = (carbohydrate calories/100 g divided by total calories) x 100 = % ME

From Case, L.P., Carey, D.P., Hirakawa, D.A., & Daristotle, L. 2000. Nutrient content of pet foods. In *Canine and feline nutrition: A resource for companion animal professionals* (2nd. ed., pp. 165-186). St. Louis, MO: Mosby.

be used. Because you are not accounting for metabolic or fecal/urine losses, these values are not as accurate as the metabolizable energy values.

By converting the nutrients into percentage of metabolizable energy, we can compare dry foods to canned foods by any manufacturer. This is the most accurate way to compare foods. It will also allow us the best way to find a food that meets a specific nutrient profile (i.e., low fat).

TABLE 12.3 **Energy density from guaranteed analysis.**

Percentage in diet of nutrient × mod. Atwater factor = kcal/100 g of food
Divided % nutrient by total calories to get nutrient distribution

Work Sheet Examples

No Name Dog Food Guarantee Analysis

Protein: 21%
Fat: 5%
Moisture: 12%
Insoluble fiber: 12%
Ash: 3%

Protein 21% × 3.5 = calories from protein per 100 g of food
73.5 protein calories

Fat 5% × 8.5 = calories from fat per 100 g of food
42.5 fat calories

Carbohydrate Needs to be calculated from given values, usually not provided
[(100 − (protein + fat + insoluble fiber + moisture + ash)]
Carbohydrate = [(100 − (21 + 5 + 12 + 12 + 3)] = 47% × 3.5 = calories from
carbohydrate per 100 g of food = 164.5 carbohydrate calories
Total calories = 73.5 + 42.5 + 164.5 = 280.5 kcal/100 g

Metabolizable Calories =

Protein 73.5/280.5 × 100 = 26.2%

Fat 42.5/280.5 × 100 = 15%

Carbohydrate 164.5/280.5 × 100 = 58.6%

From Case, L.P., Carey, D.P., Hirakawa, D.A., & Daristotle, L. 2000. Nutrient content of pet
foods. In *Canine and feline nutrition: A resource for companion animal professionals* (2nd.
ed., pp. 165–186). St. Louis, MO: Mosby; and Hand, M.S., Thatcher, C.D., & Remillard, R.I.
2000. Small animal clinical nutrition: An iterative process. In M. S. Hand, C.D. Thatcher, R.L.
Remillard, & P. Roudebush (eds.), *Small animal clinical nutrition* (4th. ed., pp. 7–11).
Marceline, MO: Walsworth Publishing for Mark Morris Institute.

References

Case, L.P., Carey, D.P., Hirakawa, D.A., & Daristotle, L. 2000. Nutrient content
of pet foods. In *Canine and feline nutrition: A resource for companion animal
professionals* (2nd. ed., pp. 165–186). St. Louis, MO: Mosby.
Eukanuba. 2003. *Veterinary diets product reference guide* (pp. 14, 46, 57). Dayton, OH: Iams.
Hand, M.S., Thatcher, C.D., & Remillard, R.I. 2000. Small animal clinical
nutrition: An iterative process. In M. S. Hand, C.D. Thatcher, R.L. Remillard,
& P. Roudebush (eds.), *Small animal clinical nutrition* (4th. ed., pp. 7–11).
Marceline, MO: Walsworth Publishing for Mark Morris Institute.

13

Types of Pet Foods

Until the early 1900s, there were few options as to what to feed our companion animals—they ate what we ate. After the start of commercial pet food production, the available options have continued to expand at an alarming rate to encompass the current amazing variety of foods and flavors.

The majority of pet owners today feed their dogs and cats commercially prepared pet foods instead of homemade diets (Case et al., 2000). These diets are available in several forms that vary according to their processing methods, the ingredients used, and the method of preservation (Case et al., 2000). The foods can be further classified based on their nutrient content, purpose of use, the quality of the ingredients, and the water content of the diet (Burger, 1995; Case et al., 2000).

The broadest method of classification is by moisture content; these categories are dry, moist, and semimoist foods (Case et al., 2000).

Dry Pet Foods

Dry pet foods contain between 6% to 10% moisture and 90% or more dry matter (DM) (Case et al., 2000). They are generally sold in the form of kibbles, biscuits, meals, and expanded, extruded pellets (Burger, 1995; Case et al., 2000; Kelly, 1996). These may be "complete and balanced" for all life stages or designed for a specific life stage.

They may also be designed to be only a treat or snack (Burger, 1995; Case et al., 2000; Kelly, 1996).

A certain level of starch content must be included in expanded products to allow for proper processing of the product. This is generally met through the inclusion of cereals, cereal byproducts, and soy meals (Case et al., 2000). The loss of nutrients, particularly vitamins, through processing is limited because the baking or extrusion processes do not require excessive temperatures or time, and sufficient supplements are added to counterbalance processing and storage losses (Burger, 1995). Because of the low moisture content of the food, they do not contain enough water for bacterial or fungal growth and have a long shelf-life if kept in cool, dry storage conditions (Burger, 1995).

Kibbles and biscuits are prepared in much the same way, although the final shapes are different (Case et al., 2000). In both cases, the ingredients are mixed together to form a dough similar to cookie dough, which is then baked. When biscuits are made, the dough is formed or cut into desired shapes and the individual biscuits are baked like cookies (Case et al., 2000). With kibbled foods, the dough is spread onto large sheets and baked. After cooling, the large sheets are broken into bite-sized pieces and packaged (Case et al., 2000). Most dog and cat treats are baked biscuits, although a few companies still produce complete and balanced kibble (Case et al., 2000). Dry meal foods are prepared by mixing together a number of dried, flaked, and granular ingredients to form a dog and cat version of "trail mix" (Case et al., 2000; Kelly, 1996).

The development of the extrusion process by Purina in the 1950s resulted in the almost complete replacement of meals and kibbles with extruded commercial foods (Case et al., 2000). The extrusion process produces expanded pet foods and involves the mixing of all the ingredients together to form dough. This dough is then cooked under conditions of high pressure and temperature in an extruder. When the cooked dough reaches the end of the extruder (within 20 to 60 seconds), it exits through a small die. This die forces the soft product into desired shape(s), and a rotating knife cuts the forms into the desired kibble size (Case et al., 2000). The extrusion process causes rapid cooking of the starches within the product, resulting in increased digestibility and palatability. After cooling, a coating of fat or digest (a type of flavor enhancer produced by chemical or enzymatic breakdown of proteins) is usually applied to the outside of the food in a process called enrobing. The enrobing further enhances the palatability of the food. Hot air drying reduces the total moisture content to 10% or less (Case et al., 2000).

Dry foods contain a greater concentration of nutrients and energy per unit weight than do foods of higher moisture content. Because of this, relatively small amounts are needed to provide a particular quantity of nutrients (Burger, 1995; Kelly, 1996). Unless the dry food contains a large amount of nondigestible fiber, the digestibility is good but often lower than that of meats or canned foods (Burger, 1995). Dry foods are considered to be better digested by dogs than by cats due to the higher carbohydrate content found in the diets (Burger, 1995). Dry foods also tend to be less expensive than canned or semimoist diets, but this can vary based on the ingredients used and the quality of those ingredients (Kelly, 1996). The primary disadvantage of dry diets is that they are less palatable than meats or canned diets (Burger, 1995). The major advantages are cost and convenience.

Most popular or premium brands of dry foods may be lower in digestible fiber than less expensive brands and are comparable to quality canned foods in digestibility of nutrients (Kelly, 1996). The stools produced will help to indicate the quality of the food—with a high-quality food, well-formed, firm stools are produced once or twice a day, whereas a poor-quality food may result in bulky, less-formed stools produced more often (Kelly, 1996).

The availability of essential fatty acids (EFAs), especially linoleic acid for the dog and arachidonic acid for the cat, can be affected by prolonged storage in less-than-optimal conditions for some complete dry foods. This would include those foods stored in warm, damp environments (kitchens) or exposed to sunlight. This is a particular problem if beef tallow (fat) is used as the fat source (Case et al., 2000; Kelly, 1996). This can also be seen in those situations where food is bought in bulk, especially to feed a small dog or cat, and stored in an open container in the kitchen for prolonged periods (6 months or longer) (Case et al., 2000; Kelly, 1996).

Moist Pet Foods

Moist diets are no longer available just in "cans"; they also come in plastic trays, foil containers, plastic cans, and pouches. All of these products have a moisture range of 72% to 85% on an "as-fed" basis (Kelly, 1996). Canned diets can be either "complete and balanced" or designed to be used for supplemental feeding, such as a treat (Case et al., 2000).

Moist diets are prepared by first blending the meat and fat ingredients with measured amounts of water. Measured amounts of dry ingredients are then added and the entire mixture is heated (Case et al., 2000). Canning occurs on a conveyer line. After filling, the cans are sealed, washed, and labeled. Pressure sterilization of canned products is called retorting (Case et al., 2000). Temperatures and times can vary with the product and can size but typically are 250 °C for 60 minutes (Case et al., 2000). After exiting the retort, the cans are cooled under controlled conditions to ensure sterility of the food and integrity of the sealed product. After cooling, paper labels are applied (Case et al., 2000).

For processing methods, there are three main types of moist foods: loaf, chunks or chunks in gravy, and a chunk-in-loaf combination (Table 13.1) (Case et al., 2000).

Depending on the ingredients used, these products can vary greatly in nutrient content, digestibility, and nutrient availability (Case et al., 2000). Many owners assume that the "meaty chunks" found in the food are indeed meat; more commonly, these chunks are textured soy product (TSP), similar to tofu. These chunks provide the owners with the visual appeal that they are looking for while keeping the cost down for the manufacturer (Case et al., 2000).

Moist diets tend to be more palatable and digestible than many dry foods, but a poor-quality moist diet would not be more digestible than a good-quality dry food (Case et al., 2000). The high heat and pressure used in processing moist diet kill harmful bacteria and cause some nutrient losses (Case et al., 2000). Manufacturers that conduct feeding trials adjust their formulas to compensate for these losses. Companies that use the calculation method to substantiate their label claims are not required to compensate for losses because the calculation method is used before processing (Case et al., 2000).

The high moisture content of these foods affects the nutrient density, meaning that these foods have less nutrients per 100 g of food that do other food types, so that food must be eaten to satisfy energy and nutrient needs (Kelly, 1996). The most palatable diets are those that contain little or no cereal products and are presented as meaty or fishy chunks

TABLE 13.1. **Types of moist food.**

Loaf	Ground cereal and chopped meat, fish, poultry. Has a solid meatloaf-like appearance
Chunks, chunks in gravy	Ground cereal and chopped or pre-formed meat. May be meat-based, fish-based or meat & cereal based. May appear as balls, shapes or chunks together with gelling agents and mineral/vitamin supplements in gravy or jelly.
Chunk-in-loaf	A combination of the chopped loaf appearance and the chunks in gravy foods.

in gravy or jelly (Burger, 1995). Protein content can range from 7% to 9% in dog foods and from 8% to 11% in cat foods on an "as-fed" basis (Burger, 1995). Digestibility of moist foods for both dogs and cats is high, being 80% to 85% for most nutrients in quality products (Burger, 1995). Energy density is highest in moist diets on a DM basis of all commercially available diets. Palatability is directly related to the meat content, with the foods higher in cereal being less palatable (Burger, 1995).

Moist foods offer extremely long shelf-life with high acceptability by the pet. Because of their nutrient content and texture, canned foods tend to be highly palatable, and if fed free choice to an animal with low energy requirements, they can override the animal's tendency to eat to meet energy requirements, resulting in overeating and obesity (Case et al., 2000). Because they are sterilized using steam and heat, no other preservatives are needed. This makes them ideal for a client concerned about the use of preservatives in their pets' food.

Not all moist foods are complete and balanced; many are designed to be used for supplemental feeding only. Many clients use these foods to "top dress" their pets' dry foods to improve palatability. This use is what they are supposed to be used for, but many animals, especially cats, can easily develop "fixed food preferences" and will only eat this one food item and refuse all others irregardless of nutrient balance (cats are not very good at math) (Case et al., 2000).

Semimoist Foods

A third class of food product is the semimoist or soft-moist foods. These foods generally contain between 15% to 30% water and can include fresh or frozen animal tissues, cereal grains, fats, and simple sugars as their main ingredients (Case et al., 2000). Semimoist foods more closely resemble dry foods in nutrient content; they do tend to have higher proportions of animal protein and a higher energy density on a DM basis (Burger, 1995). The carbohydrate portion of the diet is mainly disaccharides (sucrose) (Burger, 1995). Digestibility can be as high as 80% to 85%.

Preservation is achieved through the use of humectants and certain preservatives (Burger, 1995; Case et al., 2000). Humectants such as sugars, salts, and glycerol are included in the foods to decrease the availability of water for use by invading organisms (Burger, 1995; Case et al., 2000). This helps to retard microbial spoilage. The addition of potassium sorbate is used to inhibit the growth of yeast and molds, and small amounts of organic acids can be included to decrease the pH and further help in inhibiting bacterial growth (Burger, 1995; Case et al., 2000).

The high sugar content of many semimoist products contributes to the palatability and digestibility of these products, especially for dogs. Cats are less likely to select a sweet food than are dogs (Case et al., 2000). Semimoist diets that contain high levels of simple carbohydrates have digestibility similar to those of moist products, although because of their lower fat content the energy density tends to be lower (Case et al., 2000). The carbohydrate content of semimoist diets is similar to that found in dry food diet, but the carbohydrate type found is largely in the form of simple carbohydrates, with relatively small proportions of starch and complex carbohydrates (Case et al., 2000). Because of the use of simple carbohydrates for preservation, these diets would not be recommended for use by diabetic animals, and the use of semimoist treats should be limited to less than 10% of the overall diet.

Semimoist foods do not require refrigeration prior to use and have a relatively long shelf-life. The overall cost of the foods tends to be between that of dry foods and that of moist foods (Case et al., 2000). Because semimoist foods are usually sold in single-serving packets, though, the price is usually closer to that of moist diets (Case et al., 2000).

On an "as-fed" basis, semimoist diets have the highest caloric density compared with dry or moist diets. They have lower moisture content than do canned foods and fewer air pockets than do extruded products (Case et al., 2000).

Snacks and Treats

Snacks and treats have become increasingly popular with pet owners in recent years. Snacks and treats are usually not purchased for their nutritional value but as a way of showing love and affection for the dog or cat. Many pet owners also use snacks and treats as training aids to reinforce positive behaviors and as an aid to proper dental health (Case et al., 2000). In general, most pet owners buy treats for emotional reasons.

Because of this emotional connection, palatability is of chief importance (Case et al., 2000). In the early years, all dog treats were in the form of baked biscuits. Since the buying of treats is usually an impulse buy on the owner's part and intended as a means of showing affection or as a training aid, the design is geared primarily to the owner. Today treats can be categorized into four basic types: semimoist, biscuits, jerky, and rawhide products. Cat treats are usually in the form of either semimoist or biscuit products, with dogs preferring rawhide and jerky treats (Case et al., 2000).

Although treats and snacks do not have to be nutritionally complete, a significant proportion of the products are formulated to be complete and balanced, and some may carry the same nutritional claim as dog and cat foods (Case et al., 2000). In general, treats and snacks are highly palatable and cost significantly more than other types of pet foods when compared on a weight basis (Case et al., 2000). A large proportion of this cost is due to the larger amounts of money directed toward marketing (Case et al., 2000).

References

Burger, I.H. 1995. Balanced diets for dogs and cats. In I.H. Burger (ed.), *The Waltham book of companion animal nutrition* (pp. 52–55). Oxford: Butterworth-Heinemann.

Case, L.P., Carey, D.P., Hirakawa, D.A., & Daristotle, L. 2000. Types of pet foods. In *Canine and feline nutrition: A resource for companion animal professionals* (2nd. ed., pp. 187-197). St. Louis, MO: Mosby.

Kelly, N.C. 1996. Food types and evaluation. In N.C. Kelly & J.M. Wills (eds.), *Manual of companion animal nutrition and feeding* (pp. 22–42, 1995). Ames, IA: Iowa State Press.

14

Raw Food Diets: Fact versus Fiction

It is generally accepted that dogs were domesticated from wolves; the period of this evolution ranges from 10,000 to 135,000 years ago. Accordingly, some recent DNA research shows that this occurred in stages in different areas and that not all dog breeds came from the same wolf or from the same geographic area (Derr, 2004). The primary ancestor of the domestic cat is believed to the African wild cat, *Felis libyca*. Domestication started for cats much later than it did for dogs, about 8,000 years ago, with full domestication taking place only 4,000 years ago (Case, 2003). The time difference is reflective in what these animals were domesticated for—dogs were hunters, and cats were vermin killers on the farms. As we evolved from a hunting society to a farming society, our needs also changed.

With this history in mind, we need to look at what food these animals have consumed since they joined us in our homes. Dogs did not continue to hunt and eat raw foods once domesticated; they primarily ate our leftovers and scraps. Because we have not consumed a raw food diet since fire was discovered, our dogs did not eat raw food either. Because cats were domesticated for their ability to control small vermin, they have continued to eat a raw food diet for a much longer period of time.

Myth: Raw Food Diets Are Nutritionally Superior to Processed Diets and Are "What Nature Intended Dogs and Cats to Eat"

There is no scientific evidence showing that raw food diets are nutritionally superior to processed foods. All processed foods are required to conform to Association of American Feed Control Officials (AAFCO) standards for sale in the United States. These standards can be met in one of two ways. The food can be "formulated" to meet AAFCO standards, or feeding trials can be done. Feeding trials are the preferred method of substantiating AAFCO certification (Roudebush et al., 2000). This takes into account not only nutrient content but also nutrient loss due to processing and digestibility.

Raw food diets overall are not marketed as "complete and balanced" and therefore do not need to meet AAFCO standards. Some of the frozen diets, however, are marketed as "complete and balanced" and have AAFCO statements on the labels but have not undergone feeding trials. The claim is that these diets are "complete and balanced" over a period of time but not for each meal. There are three main types of raw food diets:

- Commercially available complete raw food diets
  - These diets are intended to be complete and balanced without the need for additional supplements. They are typically sold in frozen form.
- Homemade complete raw food diets (many recipes for homemade raw food diets are available in books, in articles, and on the Internet)
  - These diets expect the owner to balance the diets out in the long term, as each meal is not in itself balanced.
- Combination diets
  - These consist of commercially available mixes of grains and supplements. This mix is in turn combined with raw meat (Freeman & Michel, 2001).

Granted, raw food diets may be nutritionally superior to some commercially processed foods, such as poor-quality foods that have not gone through feeding trials, use lower-grade ingredients, and have high cereal contents. Feeding any premium quality food would show an improvement just due to the increased quality of the ingredients used.

Because raw food diets have not gone through feeding trials, it is difficult to know if they are nutritionally balanced. One study has looked at the nutrient content of a variety of raw food diets, both home prepared and commercially available. None of the diets studied were balanced, and all had nutrient deficiencies or excesses. These deficiencies and excesses may have been balanced out in the long term, but this is not guaranteed (Freeman & Michel, 2001).

Pet food manufacturers know what changes occur with their foods with the various processing methods and supplement as needed to maintain optimum nutrient levels. As with any science, we continue to discover every day new ways to use diet to modulate various disease or conditions—and the manufacturers continue to change and improve their foods.

Myth: Domesticated Species Tolerate Bacterial Contamination in Food without Problems, Even If They Are Pediatric, Geriatric, or Critically Ill Animals

There is no scientific evidence to support this claim, and in fact three studies have found either bacterial contamination in the food or dishes or death related to pathogenic bacteria directly related to the diet being fed (Freeman & Michel, 2001; LeJeune & Hancock, 2001; Stiver et al., 2003).

The study looking at nutrient content of the diets also looked at microbial analyses. One of the five diets yielded growth of *Escherichia coli* O157:H7 (Freeman & Michel, 2001). This strain of *E. coli* has been connected to *E. coli* infection in people and is one of the more pathogenic strains.

Another study presented in the *Journal of the American Animal Hospital Association* reported that two cats presenting for necropsy had died from septic salmonellosis. In one of the cases, salmonellosis was directly traced back to the raw food diet that had been fed. The two cases occurred 9 months apart in presentation, but the cats were from the same household. Healthy adult cats appear to have high immunologic resistance to the development of clinical salmonellosis. Cats that are immunocompromised or otherwise ill would be at increased risk of infection due to contaminated foodstuffs (Stiver et al., 2003).

Animals that are not sick themselves can also pose a public health concern due to shedding of bacteria into the environment. There are a number of bacteria that can be found on raw meat and transmitted to animals and subsequently to their owners or others in contact with the animal or their stool.

From 20% to 25% of poultry carcasses intended for human consumption test positive for *Salmonella* organisms; the raw meat used for feeding dogs is even more frequently contaminated. Most raw poultry is also contaminated with *Campylobacter* species, primarily *Campylobacter jejuni*, so food-borne infection is highly probable for dogs fed raw chicken.

Shiga toxin *E. coli* strains are routinely isolated from fresh ground hamburger. *E. coli* O157 has been identified in dog feces.

Yersinia enterocolitica can frequently be isolated from raw meat, especially pork. As much as 89% of the commercially available raw meats may be contaminated with this organism.

Numerous food-borne parasitic infections can also affect dogs and cats. Feeding raw fish can result in infection with a variety of organisms, including *Diphyllobothrium latum*, the fish tapeworm; *Opisthorchis tenuicollis*, a trematode that infects the bile duct, pancreatic ducts, and small intestines; *Dioclophyme renale*, the giant kidney worm; and *Nanophyetus salmincola*, the vector for *Neorickettsia helminthoeca*, the agent responsible for salmon poisoning disease (SPD) in dogs (LeJeune & Hancock, 2001).

Dogs routinely fed raw meat are commonly infected with the protozoan *Sarcocystis* spp., and infected dogs may excrete sporocysts in their feces and contaminate the environment. Dogs can become infected with *Toxocara canis* and with the raccoon ascarid *Baylisascaris proconis* as a result of eating raw meat. Infected dogs can develop enteritis and shed infective eggs into the environment. In humans, these two parasites cause visceral larval migrans. Dogs are also susceptible to infection with *Trichenella spiralis*, whose larvae in found encysted in meat. Undercooked or raw pork is occasionally contaminated with this parasite (LeJeune & Hancock, 2001).

Myth: Raw Food Diets Improve the Health of Pets

The primary claim from raw food proponents is that this diet improves the health of their pets. While this is fairly nebulous and hard to prove, very few medical conditions can be directly traced back to nutrition.

On average, a wolf in the wild survives only to 8 years old, but wolves in captivity can survive up to 16 years. Most deaths are attributed to predation, disease, and starvation. As Darwin showed us, life in the wild is survival of the fittest. An animal with many of the diseases we treat for commonly in small animal medicine would not survive in the wild. That, to our pets, would be the benefit of domestication. Until fairly recently, we did not have the medical knowledge to treat these conditions either, but as human medicine progresses, so does veterinary medicine.

It would be presumptuous to think that the conditions that we see and treat our cats and dogs for do not exist in the wild and that this is solely due to the diet they consume. Furthermore, what would be the hunting ability of many of our current breeds? Could a Persian administer a cervical bite to a mouse, or is their breeding-induced malocclusion too severe to do this? What are the chances that a Yorkie would be able to catch and kill anything to eat, and considering the variety of foreign objects that a Labrador eats, would it be able to find the right food to kill and eat?

Myth: Uncooked Food Is More Easily Digested because It Contains Enzymes that Cooking Destroys

Some nutrients are destroyed by heat, but not all heat-sensitive nutrients are eliminated during cooking. This is dependent on what the nutrient content of the food was initially and how the food is processed, stored, and cooked (Jones, 2003).

Heat can also affect proteins. Proteins can be "denatured." Their physical and chemical properties can be changed or altered. This happens with egg whites when they are cooked—the albumin becomes denatured and easier for the body to digest. Some proteins in meat also exist as enzymes; proponents of raw food diets contend that these enzymes become inactive when the meat is cooked. These proteins would also become inactive in the stomach when they meet up with the digestive enzymes. There are also other enzymes that are resistant to digestion (digestive enzymes) and may or may not be affected by stomach acid or heat from cooking. For the enzymes that are affected by heat, there is little evidence to suggest that they are more beneficial to animals that eat them raw (Jones, 2003).

Due to the cellulose layer found in all plant-based compounds, digestibility of these nutrients is difficult until the cellulose layer is broken down. This can be accomplished through chewing, grinding of the food, or cooking. Plant-based materials are the primary source of carbohydrates for the body; these carbohydrates in turn are used for glucose production. If insufficient carbohydrates are available for energy, the body can also use glucogenic amino acids or glycerol from fats. If adequate dietary carbohydrates are not available, amino acids will be directed away from muscle growth, fetal growth, and milk production to be used for glucose production (Roudebush et al., 2000).

As carbohydrates are heated or cooked with water, the starch contained within the cells undergoes a process called gelatinization. The greater the degree of gelatinization, the greater is the degree of digestibility. The central nervous system and the red blood cells require glucose for their energy needs. Glucose consumed in excess of energy needs can be stored as glycogen. After glycogen stores are filled, any extra carbohydrates are converted into long-chain fatty acids and stored as fat (Roudebush et al., 2000).

Because feeding trials have not been done on the majority of raw food diets, their nutrient content, digestibility, and supplementation levels are for the most part unknown. By using raw meats, clients are leaving their pets and themselves open to bacterial and parasitic infection from possibly tainted meats. And there is no guarantee of improved health; what options are available to us in treating these pets?

First and foremost, do not ostracize these clients; most people opting to feed a raw food diet are conscientious owners looking to do the best thing for their pets. They unfortunately do not have a veterinary nutritionist in their kitchens. Most important, try to get them to cook the food being fed to their pet—this will at least address the bacterial and parasitic problems. Find out what they do not like about commercially available diets; if they are misinformed on any issues, gently guide them in the right direction. If clients insist on continuing to feed raw food diets or homemade cooked diets, recommend two to four yearly visits for complete physical examinations and blood screens to detect any problems before they become severe.

References

Case, L.P. 2003. *Domestication in the cat: Its behavior, nutrition and health* (p. 7). Ames, IA: Blackwell Publishing.

Derr, M. May 20, 2004. DNA identifies dog breeds with 99% accuracy. *New York Times News Service*.

Freeman, L.M., & Michel, K.E. 2001. Evaluation of raw food diets for dogs. *Journal of the American Veterinary Medical Association, 218,* 705–709.

Jones, A.K. 2003. The great raw meat debate. *Veterinary Technician Magazine*, October, 714–715.

LeJeune, J.T., & Hancock, D.D. 2001. Public health concerns associated with feeding raw meat diets to dogs. *Journal of the American Veterinary Medical Association, 219,* 1222–1224.

Roudebush, P., Dzanis, D.A., Debraekeleer, J., & Brown, R.G. 2000. Pet food labels. In M.S. Hand, C.D. Thatcher, R.L. Remillard, & P. Roudebush (eds.), *Small animal clinical nutrition* (4th. ed., p. 1010). Marceline, MO: Walsworth Publishing for Mark Morris Institute.

Stiver, S.L., Frazier, K.S., Mauel, M.J., & Styer, E.L. 2003. Septicemic salmonellosis in two cats fed a raw meat diet. *Journal of the American Animal Hospital Association, 39,* 538–542.

15

Pet Food Preservatives

Preservatives are added to pet foods to protect nutrients from oxidative or microbial damage under normal use and storage conditions (Case et al., 2000; Hand et al., 2000; Roudebush, 1993). In general, additives other than vitamins and minerals are found in the smallest amounts in moist foods and most often are in the largest quantities in dry foods, semimoist foods, treats, and snacks (Roudebush, 1993).

Food manufacturers are responsible for ensuring that their foods remain free from bacterial contamination and harmful toxins and are protected from nutrient loss during storage (Case et al., 2000).

Foods that have no added antioxidant preservatives at the time of processing may contain ingredients such as animal fat, fish meal, and

TABLE 15.1. **Methods of preservation.**

Dry foods	Low moisture content helps to inhibit growth of most organisms.
Moist foods	Heat sterilization and anaerobic environment kill all microbes.
Semimoist foods	Low pH and humectants bind water in the food, making it unavailable to bacteria and fungi.
Frozen foods	Food is protected by storage conditions and low temperatures.
Irradiated foods	Food is sterilized by radiation.

From Case, L.P., Carey, D.P., Hirakawa, D.A., & Daristotle, L. 2000. Additives and preservatives. In *Canine and feline nutrition: A resource for companion animal professionals* (2nd. ed., pp. 180–185). St. Louis, MO: Mosby.

fat-soluble vitamins that are preserved with antioxidants (Dodds & Donoghue, 1994).

The primary nutrients that require protection during storage are fat in the form of vegetable oil or animal fat and the fat-soluble vitamins A, D, E, and K (Case et al., 2000). It takes as little as 0.05% of the fat to react with oxygen to produce rancidity (Dodds & Donoghue, 1994). Oxidation of fats results in loss of calorie content and formation of toxic forms of peroxides that can be harmful to health (Case et al., 2000). Antioxidants do not reverse the effect of oxidation once it has started, but they retard the oxidative process and prevent further destruction of fats. Therefore, to be fully effective, they must be included in the diet when it is initially mixed and processed (Dodds & Donoghue, 1994). Ingestion of inadequately preserved rancid fats may be more harmful to the health of the pet than any adverse effects of the preservatives (Dodds & Donoghue, 1994).

Food-borne infections can be caused by microorganisms such as *Escherichia coli* and species of *Salmonella, Neorickettsia, Vibrio, Yersinia,* and *Campylobacter.* Illness can also be caused by ingestion of the toxins produced by such microorganisms as *Clostridium botulinum, Bacillus cereus, Staphylococcus aureus,* and mycotoxins (Hand et al., 2000). Properly preserved foods kill most microorganisms by cooking/sterilization and prevent the proper conditions for growth.

Naturally Derived Antioxidants

Naturally derived antioxidants are commonly found in certain grains, vegetable oils, and some herbs and spices (Case et al., 2000). These antioxidants have been processed to make them more available for use (Case et al., 2000).

Mixed tocopherols, incorrectly called vitamin E, are obtained primarily from distilling soybean oil residue. Further processing separates out the α (alpha), δ (delta), and γ (gamma) fractions. Alpha-tocopherol, accurately called vitamin E, is the most biologically active form but provides little protection against oxidation in foods. Delta- and gamma-tocopherols have lower biologic activity than alpha-tocopherol but are more effective as antioxidants (Case et al., 2000). Mixed tocopherols using both alpha- and delta-tocopherols are the most effective naturally derived antioxidants and show the greatest efficacy in protecting fats in pet foods (Case et al., 2000). Because tocopherols rapidly decompose as they protect fats from oxidation, the shelf-life of foods preserved with tocopherols alone is shorter than that of foods stabilized with a mix of several different antioxidants (Case et al., 2000).

Ascorbic acid, more commonly called vitamin C, functions as an antioxidant by scavenging oxygen; however, it is water soluble and not easily mixed with the fat found in foods. It does work synergistically with other antioxidants such as the mixed tocopherols and buylated hydroxytoluene (BHT) and is included in foods for this reason (Case et al., 2000).

Ascorbyl palmitate is similar in structure to ascorbic acid but is not normally found in nature. It undergoes hydrolysis to form ascorbic acid and the fatty acid palmitic acid, both of which are found in nature. Citric acid is often used in combination with other naturally derived antioxidants (Case et al., 2000).

Dried leaves from the shrub *Rosemarius officinalis* (common rosemary) are used to make a refined extract (rosemaric acid/rosemarequinone). The extract is used to avoid the influence of the herb on the taste and odor of the food (Case et al., 2000; Hand et al., 2000). This extract is effective in high-fat diets and has been shown to enhance the antioxidant efficiency when included in combination with mixed tocopherols, ascorbic acid, and citric acid (Case et al., 2000).

Lecithin, modified starches, monoglycerides, and diglycerides are naturally derived compounds that act as emulsifying agents, preventing separation of fats from other dietary components and allowing greater contact between antioxidants and fats (Case et al., 2000).

Potassium sorbate is used to prevent the formation of yeast and molds in foods. Glycerol and certain other sugars are used as humectants to keep foods soft and moist (Case et al., 2000).

Effective antioxidants must have good carry-through. This is the retention of antioxidant functions after being subjected to the high heat, pressure, and moisture of pet food processing (Case et al., 2000). Because most naturally derived antioxidants have poor carry-through, excessive amounts must be included to compensate for the high losses that occur during processing (Case et al., 2000). Naturally derived preservatives tend to be significantly more expensive than synthetic ones, so it is difficult to achieve necessary levels of protection using only naturally derived products without production being cost prohibitive (Case et al., 2000).

Synthetic Antioxidants

Synthetic antioxidants are made in laboratories and not from naturally derived products. The U.S. Food and Drug Administration (FDA) has approved butylated hydroxyanisole (BHA) and BHT for use in both human and animal foods. They have a synergistic antioxidant effect when used together and exhibit good carry-through and increased efficiency compared with naturally derived antioxidants in protecting animal fats but have slightly lower efficacy in protecting vegetable oils (Case et al., 2000).

Tertiary butylhydroquinine (TBHQ) is an effective antioxidant for most fats and is approved for human and animal use in the United States. However, TBHQ has not been approved for use in Canada, Japan, or the European Union, so it is not used in foods for the international market (Case et al., 2000).

Ethoxyquin is approved for use in human and animal foods and has been in use for over 30 years (Case et al., 2000; Dzanis, 1991). Its mechanism of action is similar to those of BHA and BHT in that it reduces oxidative damage of polyunsaturated fatty acids, vitamins A and E, and other fat-soluble substances by stopping free radical formation (Dzanis, 1991). Ethoxyquin is more efficient that either BHA or BHT in protecting oils with high levels of polyunsaturated fatty acids such as linoleic, alpha-linolenic, and arachidonic acids. This allows for lower levels of antioxidants to be added to the final product (Dzanis, 1991).

Ethoxyquin has a toxicity rating of 3 and is considered to be moderately toxic. This rating is slightly higher than that for tetracycline or penicillin and is lower than that for aspirin or caffeine (Dodds & Donoghue, 1994). Ethoxyquin is readily absorbed, metabolized, and excreted in the urine and feces. Residual levels are found in the liver, gastrointestinal tract, and adipose tissue (Dodds & Donoghue, 1994). Before ethoxyquin gained FDA approval, the manufacturer (Monsanto, St. Louis, MO) conducted a 1-year chronic toxicity study in dogs in which "no observable effect level" was determined to be 3 mg/kg administered on a 5 day/week schedule (Dzanis, 1991). Mild changes were seen histopathologically in the liver and kidneys at much higher doses (10 mg/kg), with more pronounced signs of toxicity observed at 50 and 100 mg/kg (Dzanis, 1991). The FDA Center for Veterinary Medicine requested as of July 31, 1997, that manufacturers voluntarily lower the maximum level of ethoxyquin in complete dog food to 75 parts per million (ppm) from the allowed 150 ppm to further increase the margin of safety for lactating females and puppies (personal communication, August 1997, FDA Center for Veterinary Medicine).

Ethoxyquin and other synthetic preservatives have been blamed for widespread infertility; neonatal illness and death; skin and coat problems; immune disorders; dysfunction of the thyroid, liver, and pancreas; and behavioral problems (Dzanis, 1991; Hand et al., 2000; Roudebush, 1993). Reports of adverse reactions have been almost exclusively in dogs, the majority of these being purebred or inbred animals (Dzanis,

TABLE 15.2.　Characteristics of some antioxidants.

Antioxidant	Carry-through	Effectiveness
Naturally derived		
Mixed tocopherols	Poor	Low
Ascorbic acid	Poor	Low
Ascorbyl palmitate	Poor	Low
Synthetic		
Butylated hydroxyanisole	Good	High
Butylated hydrosytoluene	Good	High
Tertiary butylhydroquine	Good	High
Ethoxyquin	Excellent	High

From Case, L.P., Carey, D.P., Hirakawa, D.A., & Daristotle, L. 2000. Additives and preservatives. In *Canine and feline nutrition: A resource for companion animal professionals* (2nd. ed., pp. 180–185). St. Louis, MO: Mosby.

1991; Roudebush, 1993). To date, the FDA had found no scientific or medical evidence that ethoxyquin used at approved levels is injurious to human or animal health (Hand et al., 2000). After gaining FDA approval for ethoxyquin, Monsanto conducted an additional study of a multigenerational group of dogs over a 5-year period using foods with two times the approved level of ethoxyquin at that time (i.e., 300 ppm) (Dzanis, 1991). No adverse effects, especially those noted by breeders, were found in these dogs.

Need for Preservatives

The need for antioxidants in pet foods is obvious. Therefore, questions about the safety of preservatives need to be balanced against the needs of the pets. Canned or frozen foods have the lowest levels of antioxidants because they are preserved by either heat or cold, not by antioxidants. Some pet food manufacturers produce dry foods that are preserved with naturally derived antioxidants, although they may contain small amounts of synthetic antioxidants in the vitamin premix. When buying a food preserved with only naturally derived antioxidants, look for a "best if used by" date, and use the food within this time frame. If no date is included on the package label, contact the manufacturer for information on when the product was manufactured and its shelf-life.

The FDA requires that preservatives in quantities high enough to affect the final product must be listed on food labels. If the preservative is present in trivial amounts or no longer serves a technical or functional effect, it may be exempt from inclusion on the label (D. Dzanis, personal communication to Dr. Katherine Michel, University of Pennsylvania, regarding FDA labeling requirements for antioxidants, March 21, 2001). This applies to premixes or vitamin additives in foods. Ethoxyquin is an exception to this regulation; the FDA Center for Veterinary Medicine has stated that ethoxyquin should be declared on labeling regardless of the source or final level in the food (D. Dzanis, personal communication to Dr. Katherine Michel, March 21, 2001).

Manufacturers of premium pet foods conduct feeding trials on their products to detect deficiencies or other problems before foods are released for sale. Check labels to see whether feeding trials have been done. Manufacturers must state how they have met Association of American Feed Control Officials (AAFCO) standards. The label should also list all the ingredients from the largest amount to the smallest.

References

Case, L.P., Carey, D.P., Hirakawa, D.A., & Daristotle, L. 2000. Additives and preservatives. In *Canine and feline nutrition: A resource for companion animal professionals* (2nd. ed., pp. 180–185). St. Louis, MO: Mosby.

Dodds, W.J., & Donoghue, S. 1994. Interactions of clinical nutrition with genetics. In Wills, J.M., & Simpson, K.W. (eds.), *Waltham Book of clinical nutrition in the dog and ca* (pp. 114–115). Tarrytown, NY; Pergamon Press.

Dzanis, D. 1991. Safety of ethoxyquin in dog foods. *Journal of Nutrition, 121,* S163–S164.

Hand, M., Hatcher, C., Remillard, R., & Roudebush, P. 2000. Preservatives, antioxidants and contaminants: Food-borne illness. In M.S. Hand, C.D. Thatcher, R.L. Remillard, & P. Roudebush (eds.), *Small animal clinical nutrition* (4th. ed., pp. 31–33). Marceline, MO: Walsworth Publishing for Mark Morris Institute.

Roudebush, P. 1993. Food additives. *Journal of the American Medical Association, 203,* 1667–1670.

16

Homemade Diets

Counseling clients on feeding is one of the most important client education areas that the veterinary team can offer (Strombeck, 1999b). Even though the majority of pet owners in the United States enjoy the convenience, economy, and reliability of commercially produced diets, some owners still prefer to prepare homemade diets for their pets (Case et al., 2000). The reasons that clients choose to feed a home-prepared diet vary greatly; the following are some of the most common reasons (Kelly, 1996; Remillard et al., 2000):

- Clients adopt a traditional approach, being among a minority of owners not using commercially prepared food.
- Food preference has been induced in pets by exposure to home-cooked food from kittenhood or puppyhood.
- Anthropomorphism gives human food preferences to pets.
- Finicky eaters will "hold out" for tasty home-cooked treats.
- Home-prepared "elimination diets" may work better in some food-related disease, such as skin problems.
- There is a poor owner perception of commercially prepared foods as "unwholesome" or as unappetizing.
- Client wants to feed "what nature intended."
- Veterinary therapeutic diets may lack palatability or acceptability, particularly in advanced illness.
- Clients want to be involved in the care of their pet, especially older or ill animals.

- Owners wish to use ingredients that are fresh, wild grown, organic, or natural.
- There is concern that the ingredient list is an indecipherable list of chemicals.
- Clients hope to construct a nutritional profile for dietary management of a disease for which no commercial food is available.
- Owners wish to provide food variety as a defense against malnutrition, or because of the popular idea that animals need variety.
- Owners wish to lower feeding costs through the use of significant quantities of table foods and leftovers.
- Owners wish to feed a pet according to human nutritional guidelines such as a low-fat or low-cholesterol diet.
- The clients want to feed their pet according to their diet preferences, such as vegetarian diets.

When clients want to feed homemade diets, it is important to understand the reasons and motivations. In many cases it is possible to address their concerns and to recommend an appropriate commercial diet that will meet everyone's needs (Remillard et al., 2000). In those instances where a client is insistent about cooking for their pet, it is always better to provide them with a well-designed homemade recipe rather than allowing them to prepare food according to their own or a breeder's well-intentioned formulation that may have significant nutrient excesses and deficiencies (Remillard et al., 2000).

Any ingredients used in homemade diets should be fit for human consumption. The quality of the nutrients depends on the source and digestibility (Kelly, 1996). One of the problems with preparing homemade diets is that many of the recipes that are available have not been adequately tested for nutrient content and availability (Case et al., 2000). Poor feeding management, rather than faulty diets, is believed to be responsible for many nutritional problems (Strombeck, 1999b). Even if a balanced diet is offered, clients will usually "adjust" the ingredients to their likes, very likely upsetting any balance that the diet did have, or will supplement with treats or snacks in excess of 10% of the diet. It should be noted that the primary "malnutrition" that is seen in dogs and cats today is obesity. This would be even more likely to occur when an animal is fed a homemade, highly palatable diet with unknown nutrient density.

Food Preparation

Any food fed to a pet needs to be properly cooked before feeding. Cooking improves digestibility and kills bacteria and parasites that might cause disease (Strombeck, 1999a). However, cooking does not eliminate the problem caused by endotoxins released from dead bacteria (Strombeck, 1999a). These endotoxins can be found in meats previously contaminated by coliform bacteria (Strombeck, 1999b). Nothing can be done to decontaminate a food containing endotoxins (Strombeck, 1999a).

When foods are prepared at home, safe food handling and preparation methods determine whether the final diet will be safe for consumption (Strombeck, 1999a). Safe handling of food by owners begins at the store and continues in the home. Safe handling prevents or minimizes hazards associated with biological (bacteria), chemical (cleaning agents), and physical (equipment) causes (Strombeck, 1999a).

According to the Centers for Disease Control and Prevention (CDC), hand washing is the single most important means of preventing the spread of infection from bacteria, pathogens, and viruses causing disease and food-borne illnesses (Strombeck, 1999a). Food preparation most importantly includes hand washing done before and after handling of each ingredient in the diet (Strombeck, 1999a). In addition to hand washing, counters, equipment, utensils, and cutting boards should be sanitized with a dilute bleach solution (Strombeck, 1999a). Frozen foods should never be thawed at room temperature; thawing should be done in the refrigerator, the microwave, or a cold water bath (Strombeck, 1999a).

All ingredients used in the diet should always be cooked thoroughly. Freezing or rinsing with cold water is not an acceptable method for destroying bacteria (Strombeck, 1999a). Once a diet is cooked, it may be stored in the refrigerator and reheated later before serving (Strombeck, 1999a).

Ingredient Choices

Many owners choose their pet's diet ingredients based on their own preferences, product availability, or affordability (Remillard et al., 2000). Other pets are fed a variety of leftovers, such as fat trimmings, vegetable skins, crusts, and condiments. These diets are rarely representative of the owner's diet and are not "complete and balanced" for the pet (Remillard et al., 2000).

Owners may also choose the ingredients based on current human nutrition trends. As we know, there are several differences between canine, feline, and human nutrition, as well as nutrient digestion and needs. Those clients who choose to feed their pets vegetarian diets are at greatest risk of feeding an unbalanced, inadequate diet. There are a number of commercially prepared canine vegetarian diets that are complete and balanced (Remillard et al., 2000). Clients should be strongly discouraged from feeding cats vegetarian diets, because cats are strict carnivores. Without adequate supplementation (usually available from only meat-based products), cats fed vegetarian or vegan diets are at high risk for taurine, arginine, tryptophan, lysine, arachidonic acid, and vitamin A deficiency. These deficiencies are life threatening and can lead to the death of the cat (Remillard et al., 2000).

Due to inconvenience, expense, or failure to understand its importance, many clients eliminate the vitamin and mineral supplements in homemade diets. This would cause a recipe that was crudely balanced to become grossly imbalanced (Remillard et al., 2000).

Assess the Recipe

If able, offer the client a nutritionally adequate recipe rather than having them either make their own or use one from a nonveterinary source. Homemade formulation can be checked for nutritional adequacy and adjusted using the "quick check" guidelines below (Remillard et al., 2000):

- Do five food groups appear in the recipe?

  ○ Carbohydrate/fiber source
  ○ Protein source, preferable animal origin
  ○ Fat source
  ○ Mineral source, primarily calcium
  ○ Multivitamin and trace mineral source

- Is the carbohydrate source cooked and present in higher or equal quantity as the protein source?

  ○ Feline carbohydrate:protein, 1:1 to 2:1
  ○ Canine carbohydrate:protein, 2:1 to 3:1

- What are the type and quantity of the primary protein source?

  ○ Final food should contain 25% to 30% cooked meat for dogs and 35% to 50% cooked meat for cats. Skeletal muscle meat is preferred. Liver can be used once weekly. If feeding lacto-ovo vegetarian diets, eggs are the best protein source; if feeding a vegan diet, soybeans provide the next best protein source but has an incomplete amino acid profile (Remillard et al., 2000).

- Is the primary protein source lean or fatty?

  o If using a "lean" meat, an additional fat should be added, either animal, vegetable, or fish source.
  o 2% of the total formula weight for dogs
  o 5% of the total formula weight for cats

- Is a source of calcium and other minerals provided?

  o Absolute calcium deficiency is most common in homemade diets.
  o Milk products usually contribute inadequate amounts of calcium to diet.

- Is a source of vitamins and other nutrients provided?

  o An adult over-the-counter supplement that contains no more than 200% of the recommended daily allowances for humans usually works well for dog and cats.
  o Give ½ to 1 tablet per day, based on pet size.
  o Cats should receive additional taurine supplementation, between 200 and 500 mg/day, depending on the diet's calculated taurine content.
  o Iodized salt should be use to meet the iodine requirement (Remillard et al., 2000).

Selecting a Diet

There are software programs available to help you formulate a balanced diet from scratch, or you can contact a member of the American College of Veterinary Nutritionist (ACVN) for food recommendations; many veterinary schools also offer help with homemade recipes. In addition, there are many published recipes available—be sure to critically evaluate the source and check whether any testing has been done on the recipe. Strombeck (1999b), Kelly (1996), and Remillard et al. (2000) provide a variety of recipes as well as acceptable substitutions.

Additional Instructions

Be sure to provide specific instructions for preparation, storage, and feeding of homemade foods to the pet owners. Explain the importance of each ingredient as well as the proper proportions to be used. If owners choose to make batches of food instead of cooking daily, the food will need to be stored in airtight containers in the refrigerator or frozen until use. Foods should not be stored longer than 3 to 7 days in the refrigerator. Foods will need to be checked daily for any changes in color or odor that may indicate spoilage or deterioration (Remillard et al., 2000).

Prior to serving the food, if refrigerated or frozen, it should be warmed to slightly below body temperature. Warn clients to carefully check for "hot spots" in the food that could burn the animal's mouth (Remillard et al., 2000).

Patient Assessment and Monitoring

Dogs and cats that are fed homemade diets should be brought in to the clinic for veterinary evaluations two or three times per year. This will help to identify any problems with the diet before they become too great to fix (Remillard et al., 2000).

The effectiveness of a diet can be grossly evaluated by noting the patient's body weight, body condition, and activity level. Laboratory levels such as albumin, red blood cell number and size, and hemoglobin concentration are gross estimations of the animal's nutritional status. More specifically, the skin and hair should be examined closely, and an ophthalmic evaluation looking at the lens and retina should be performed. Stool quality also needs to be assessed (Remillard et al., 2000).

References

Case, L.P., Carey, D.P., Hirakawa, D.A., & Daristotle, L. 2000. Types of pet foods. In *Canine and feline nutrition: A resource for companion animal professionals* (2nd. ed., p. 196). St. Louis, MO: Mosby.

Kelly, N.C. 1996. Food types and evaluation. In N.C. Kelly & J.M. Wills (eds.), *Manual of companion animal nutrition and feeding* (pp. 38–41). Ames, IA: Iowa State Press.

Remillard, R.L., Paragon, B.-M., Crane, S.W., Debraekeleer, J., & Cowell, C.S. 2000. Making pet foods at home. In M.S. Hand, C.D. Thatcher, R.L. Remillard, & P. Roudebush (eds.), *Small animal clinical nutrition* (4th. ed., pp. 163–179). Marceline, MO: Walsworth Publishing for Mark Morris Institute.

Strombeck, D.R. 1999a. Food safety and preparation. In *Home-prepared dog and cat diets: The healthful alternative* (pp. 43–61). Ames, IA: Iowa State Press.

Strombeck, D.R. 1999b. Introduction. In *Home-prepared dog and cat diets: The healthful alternative* (pp. 3–19). Ames, IA: Iowa State Press.

3

Feeding Management for Dogs and Cats

17

Feeding Regimens for Dogs and Cats

To understand normal feeding behaviors in domestic dogs and cats, you first need to understand the origin of these behaviors and how they differ from those still found in the wild.

Feeding behaviors include searching, hunting, and caching of prey, as well as postprandial grooming and sleeping (Voith, 1994). An obvious difference between domestic dogs and cats and their wild ancestors is the amount of energy expended in obtaining a meal (Case et al., 2000). Wild dogs and cats expend considerable amounts of energy locating and capturing a meal, and their success is not guaranteed. They, for the most part, do not have a reliable and consistent source of food (Case et al., 2000). In an effort to maintain access to food, additional energy is expended in territorial behaviors (Voith, 1994). Our domestic pets are usually provided with a consistent source of nutritious and palatable foods, and expend only the effort required for begging to obtain this (Case et al., 2000).

Dogs

Wolves, our modern-day dogs' wild ancestor, hunt in packs, using cooperative behavior to prey on large animals that otherwise would be unavailable to an animal hunting on its own (Case et al., 2000). This cooperative behavior allows for larger amounts of food being obtained but also dictates the type of feeding behavior seen—that of gorging themselves immediately after a kill and then not eating for extended periods of time (Case et al., 2000). Food is consumed rapidly, and in a predetermined order within the pack. Any food that is left over is hoarded or cached for consumption later, when food is not so readily available (Case et al., 2000).

These gorging and hoarding behaviors can be seen in some of our domestic dogs today. This can lead to choking and swallowing of large amounts of air during eating (Case et al., 2000). Dogs may also eat more rapidly if fed in a group situation rather than alone. Changing the feeding situation can help to curb the gorging behavior; if this is occurring in a pack situation, remove the dog from the pack and feed it by itself. If the dog is consuming the food too quickly, sometimes changing the type of food offered can help, as well as changing how that food is offered. It is much easier to eat large amounts of canned food out of a bowl, than it is to eat large amounts of dry food fed off of a flat tray (Case et al., 2000).

Conversely, the presence of another dog may stimulate the appetite of a poor eater so they consume more food than if fed alone (Case et al., 2000). Dominance may also play a part in the amount of food consumed within a group, with the dominant dog eating more than its share and the subordinate dog not getting enough food to eat. Separating the dogs at meal time may help, as well as designating feeding location or bowls for each dog (Case et al., 2000).

Domestic dogs still hoard choice food items, as can be seen with buried bones in the yard and treats hidden in furniture and under beds (Case et al., 2000). Unlike their wild ancestors, domestic dogs often forget about these hidden items, leading to quite a collection in various places within the house and yard.

If we look to the wolf for our domestic dogs' feeding schedule, large meals fed infrequently would seem to be the natural way to feed (Case et al., 2000). However, when domestic dogs are given free-choice access to food, they tend to eat small meals frequently throughout the day (Case et al., 2000; Voith, 1994). This pattern is similar to that seen with cats, with the exception that dogs tend to eat only during the day (Case et al., 2000). Our domestic dogs can readily adapt to a number of feeding regimens, the primary ones being portion-controlled feeding, time-controlled feeding, and free-choice or ad libitum feeding (Case et al., 2000).

Cats

As much as domestic cats look like their wild ancestors, the tiger and lion, they are actually descendant from the much smaller African wildcat, *Felis silvestris libyca*. This distinction is important because the larger cats eat larger prey less frequently, while the smaller African wildcat consumes multiple small meals throughout the day. This leads to a more ad libitum type of feeding schedule for the smaller cats (Voith, 1994). There is no convincing evidence that the smaller cats engage in cooperative hunting behaviors, even when living in large groups (Voith, 1994). Because these cats hunt alone and consume small meals frequently, they tend to consume their meals slowly and are uninhibited by the presence of other animals (Case et al., 2000). This same type of behavior can readily be seen with our own domestic cats. If fed free choice, they will nibble at their food throughout the day and night. It is not unusual for a cat to eat between 9 and 16 meals per day, with each meal having a calorie content of about 23 kcal. Like the dog, the cat is able to adapt to a number of different feeding regimens, although time-controlled feeding with cats does not work as well as it does with dogs (Case et al., 2000).

What to Feed

As listed in previous chapters, the food choices for owners include dry, semimoist, moist, and homemade diets. Most owners prefer the convenience, cost effectiveness, and reliability of feeding commercial foods. If the choice is made to feed a homemade diet, care must be exercised to ensure that the diet is complete and balanced and that all ingredients and the final product are safe to consume and stored properly (Case et al., 2000). Surveys have shown that more than 90% of owners feed commercial foods to their pets (Case et al., 2000).

One of the most important considerations when deciding what to feed an animal is the life stage of the pet (Case et al., 2000). Nutrient and energy needs will differ according to an animal's age, activity level, reproductive status, and health (Case et al., 2000). Specific diets have been developed by commercial pet food manufacturers to address the needs of pets during different ages and physiologic states (Case et al., 2000).

When evaluating a diet to be fed, some other important considerations for all life stages are as follows (Case et al., 2000):

- Does the food provide all the essential nutrients in adequate amounts and proper balance to meet the lifestyle and life stage needs?
- Does the food supply sufficient energy to maintain ideal body condition and weight as well as support optimal tissue growth?

- Is the food palatable enough to ensure that the animal will willingly consume it over an extended period when fed as the primary diet?
- Does extended use support proper gastrointestinal function and consistently result in the production of regular, firm, well-formed stools?
- With extended use, is the animal subjectively healthy, with good coat quality, healthy skin condition, proper body physique, and muscle tone, and does the animal have sufficient energy to function as desired?

While many of these qualities are subjective and can only be assessed over an extended period of time, some of the answers can be found in the product reference guides supplied by the pet food manufacturers. Have feeding trials been done on this food? What is the life stage rating? What is the metabolizable energy of the diet? And what is the nutrient density of the diet? Many clients do not connect the quality of the diet being fed to their pet to the condition of the skin and coat, the stool quality, or the lack of endurance when exercising. If they are reluctant to follow your dietary recommendations, use the list from above to compare the diet they are currently feeding with what you are recommending.

Feeding Regimens

The three primary feeding choices available for dogs and cats are free-choice or ad libitum, time-controlled feeding, and portion-controlled or measured feeding (Case et al., 2000).

The method used will be determined by the owner's daily schedule, the number of animals being fed, the type of food being fed, and the acceptability of the method to the pet or pets (Voith, 1994).

Free-Choice Feeding

Free-choice feeding is having a surplus of food available at all times. This enables the pet or pets to consume as much food as desired at any time of the day (Case et al., 2000). This feeding method relies on the animal's ability to self-regulate food intake so that only the actual energy and nutrient needs are met, and no excess energy is consumed (Case et al., 2000). Dry food is the best choice for this method as it will not spoil or dry out as easily as other products. This does not mean that by feeding dry food, the dishes do not need to be cleaned or the food refreshed daily (Case et al., 2000).

When compared with the other methods, free-choice feeding requires the least amount of work and knowledge by the owner (Case et al., 2000). The food and water supply are replenished only once daily (or less often), and it is not necessary for the owner to determine the pet's exact daily energy requirements (Case et al., 2000). When dogs are fed free-choice, they tend to consume frequent small meals throughout the day. This feeding pattern has the advantage of greater meal-induced energy loss through digestion compared with dogs that eat larger meals and less frequently (Case et al., 2000). However, this increased energy loss is usually more than compensated for by increased energy intake by most dogs.

Free-choice feeding can be a helpful way to feed those animals that are "poor doers" and do not eat sufficient calories to support themselves when fed time-controlled meals. This allows them to eat multiple small meals throughout the day, increasing their overall energy intake. This method can also be helpful for animals that work at a very high energy level, by allowing them to replenish their energy reserves throughout the day (Case et al., 2000).

Free-choice feeding can be a disadvantage if animals are having problems with anorexia or overconsumption, as these problems may go undetected for an extended period of time (Case et al., 2000). If these problems are related to a medical condition, valuable time may be lost until the animal is sick enough for the owner to notice a change in the condition; if the animal were meal or portion fed, the problem with increased or decreased intake would be evident to the owner within a short period of time (Case et al., 2000).

Obesity is a common problem with animals that are fed free-choice food. With a highly palatable diet and a sedentary lifestyle, the normal regulatory mechanisms used to control food intake are easily overridden (Case et al., 2000). In young growing animals, this overconsumption of energy has been shown to cause an accelerated growth rate and increased fat deposition within the body, further contributing to obesity later in life (Case et al., 2000).

Time-Controlled Feeding

Time-controlled feeding involves controlling the amount of time the animal is given access to the food, but the animal can eat as much as it wants or can within this period of time (Case et al., 2000). This method also relies on the animal's ability to regulate its own energy intake. At mealtime, a surplus amount of food is supplied and the animal is allowed to eat for a predetermined period of time. For most dogs and cats that are not physiologically stressed, 15 to 20 minutes is sufficient to meet their energy requirements (Case et al., 2000). This is usually done in either one or two meals daily. While most animals can eat a sufficient amount of food when fed once daily, twice daily is healthier and more satisfying for the animal (Case et al., 2000). Twice-daily feeding will also help to reduce hunger between meals and decrease food-associated behaviors such as begging and stealing food (Case et al., 2000).

Some animals do not adapt well to time-controlled feedings. Some may not consume a sufficient quantity within the time period allotted, whereas others will gorge themselves throughout the entire period of time, leading to obesity. Time-controlled feedings may actually encourage gluttonous behavior because animals quickly learn that they have to "beat the clock" (Case et al., 2000).

Portion-Controlled Feeding

Portion-controlled feeding is the preferred method in most situations (Case et al., 2000). By feeding a predetermined amount of food once or twice daily, the owner is given the greatest amount of control over the pet's diet. Portion-controlled feedings also allow the owner to monitor the food intake more closely and notice any changes in intake or behavior quickly (Case et al., 2000). This method also allows the most control over growth rate and weight and can be adjusted as needed to maintain the desired effect (Case et al., 2000). By doing this, conditions related to overweight, underweight, or inappropriate growth can be corrected at an early stage (Case et al., 2000).

Portion-controlled feeding also demands the most amount of knowledge and effort by the owner. Guidelines for feeding amounts are provided on the bags or containers of food; these can be used as a starting point to determine the amount of food to be fed to the animal (Case et al., 2000). The daily energy requirements (DER) can also be calculated using the pet's weight and activity level and the energy density of the food. The manufacturer can be contacted to determine the energy density of the food, because this is usually not provided on the product label.

The time commitment for portion-controlled feeding is usually not a problem for most owners unless a large number of animals are being fed at any one time. The easiest method is to coordinate the pet's meal time with the owners' meal time; this would also have the added bonus of decreasing begging at the table because the pet is eating its own food (Case et al., 2000).

References

Case, L.P., Carey, D.P., Hirakawa, D.A., & Daristotle, L. 2000. Feeding regimens in dogs and cats. In *Canine and feline nutrition: A resource for companion animal professionals* (2nd. ed., pp. 217–224). St. Louis, MO: Mosby.
Voith, V.L. 1994. Feeding behaviors. In J.M. Wills & K.W. (eds.), *The Waltham book of clinical nutrition of the dog and cat* (pp. 119–127). Tarrytown, NY: Pergamon Press.

18

Body Condition Scoring

Use of the body condition score (BCS) is a subjective assessment of an animal's body fat and, to a lesser extent, protein stores (Burkholder & Toll, 2000). The scoring system takes into account the animal's frame size independent of its weight. In animals, the subcutaneous fat adheres more to muscle than to skin, making skin-fold thickness a questionable means for determining body fat in cats and dogs (Burkholder, 2000).

There are two main scoring systems—the 5-point scale and the 9-point scale. Both systems use defined criteria to help make the subjective process of body evaluation more objective, but not all subjectivity can be removed when assigning a score to an animal. For this reason, it is important that the same person try to assign the score each time the animal is evaluated. The 5-point scale scores the animals to the nearest half score, and a 9-point scale scores to the nearest whole score (Burkholder & Toll, 2000).

Studies have shown that body fat increases 5% to 7% for each whole increment increase using a 9-point scale with mid-range scoring animals (4/9 to 5/9) having 15% to 20% of their body mass as fat (Burkholder, 2000). When trying to detect small changes in body fat, the use of BCS scores would probably not be the best choice, but for monitoring and routine care, it is quick, easy, and painless.

Body Condition Score Uses

A BCS should be recorded with the weight each time an animal is examined. Body weight alone does not indicate how appropriate the weight is for the individual animal. The BCS puts in perspective what an individual animal should weigh (Burkholder & Toll, 2000).

In general, dogs and cats with an optimal body condition have:

- Normal body contours and silhouettes.
- Bony prominences that are easily palpated but not seen or felt above the skin surface.
- Intra-abdominal fat that is insufficient to obscure or interfere with abdominal palpation.

Normal BCSs are 3/5 or 4/9 to 5/9; when scores are below 2/5 or 3/9 or are above 4/5 or 7/9, then action should be taken to bring the animal into a more normal BCS (Burkholder & Toll, 2000).

TABLE 18.1.   **Five-point body condition score.**

BCS	What You See	What You Feel
1/5 Emaciated	Obvious ribs, pelvic bones and spine, no body fat or muscle mass	Bones with little covering of muscle
2/5 Thin	Ribs and pelvic bones, but less prominent; tips of spine, an "hourglass" waist (looking from above), a tucked up abdomen (looking from side)	Ribs and other bones with no palpable fat, but some muscle present
3/5 Moderate	Less prominent hourglass and abdominal tuck	Ribs without excess fat covering
4/5 Stout	General fleshy appearance, hourglass and abdominal tuck hard to see	Ribs, with difficulty
5/5 Obese	Sagging abdomen, large deposits of fat over chest, abdomen, and pelvis	Nothing, except general flesh

From Case, L.P., Carey, D.P., Hirakawa, D.A., & Daristotle, L. 2000. Adult maintenance. In *Canine and feline nutrition: A resource for companion animal professionals* (2nd. ed., pp. 256-257). St. Louis, MO: Mosby.

TABLE 18.2. **Five-point body condition score card.**

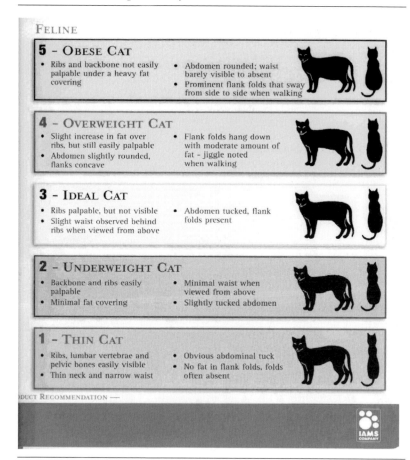

FELINE

5 - OBESE CAT
- Ribs and backbone not easily palpable under a heavy fat covering
- Abdomen rounded; waist barely visible to absent
- Prominent flank folds that sway from side to side when walking

4 - OVERWEIGHT CAT
- Slight increase in fat over ribs, but still easily palpable
- Abdomen slightly rounded, flanks concave
- Flank folds hang down with moderate amount of fat - jiggle noted when walking

3 - IDEAL CAT
- Ribs palpable, but not visible
- Slight waist observed behind ribs when viewed from above
- Abdomen tucked, flank folds present

2 - UNDERWEIGHT CAT
- Backbone and ribs easily palpable
- Minimal fat covering
- Minimal waist when viewed from above
- Slightly tucked abdomen

1 - THIN CAT
- Ribs, lumbar vertebrae and pelvic bones easily visible
- Thin neck and narrow waist
- Obvious abdominal tuck
- No fat in flank folds, folds often absent

PRODUCT RECOMMENDATION —

IAMS COMPANY

(Provided courtesy of the Iams Co., Dayton, OH.)

Just because an animal scores 5/5 or 9/9 does not mean that this is the maximum size or weight that this animal can attain. In fact, animals can be scored as a 5/5+ or 9/9+ if morbid obesity is present. There is no "maximum" amount of body fat compatible with life (Burkholder & Toll, 2000).

TABLE 18.3.   **Nine-point body condition score.**

BCS	What You See	What You Feel
1/9 Emaciated	Obvious ribs, pelvic bones, and spine, no body fat or muscle mass	Bones with little covering of muscle
2/9	Obvious ribs, pelvic bones, and spine, minimal body fat, minimal loss of muscle mass	Bones with some covering of muscle
3/9 Thin	Ribs and pelvic bones, but less prominent; an "hourglass" waist (looking from above), a tucked up abdomen (looking from side)	Ribs and other bones with no palpable fat, but more muscle present
4/9 Ideal	Minimal fat covering, waist easily seen from above, abdominal tuck evident	Ribs easily palpated, muscle mass present
5/9	Less prominent hourglass and abdominal tuck	Ribs without excess fat covering
6/9 Heavy	Slight fat covering, waist evident when viewed from above, but not prominent, abdominal tuck apparent	Ribs palpable with slight excess fat covering
7/9	General fleshy appearance, hourglass and abdominal tuck hard to see	Ribs, with difficulty, fat deposits over noticeable lumbar and at base of tail
8/9	Heavy fat deposits over lumbar area and at base of tail, waist absent, no abdominal tuck evident, obvious abdominal distention	Ribs not palpable under heavy fat cover, obvious fat deposits over lumbar and at base of tail, abdominal palpation difficult
9/9 Obese	Sagging abdomen, large deposits of fat over chest, abdomen and pelvis	Nothing, except general flesh

From Nestle Purina body condition score card (St. Louis, MO).

Using BCS is an effective means of monitoring an animal's condition as well as its weight and is something that can be easily learned by most pet owners and done at home. This should be instituted early on in the client–patient–veterinary team relationship so that obesity and all of the associated problems can be prevented.

TABLE 18.4.   Nine-point body condition score card.

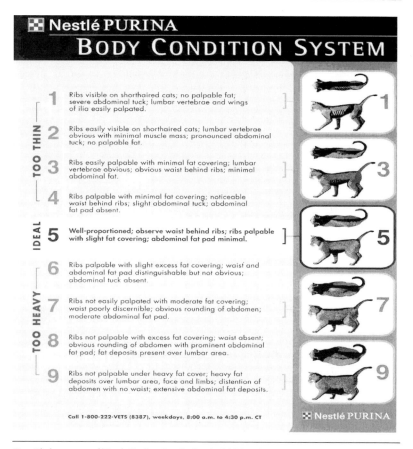

(Provided courtesy of Nestle Purina Co., St. Louis, MO.)

References

Buffington, T., Holloway, C.A., & Abood, S.K. 2004. Nutritional assessment. In *Manual of veterinary dietetics* (pp. 4–5). St. Louis, MO: Elsevier.

Burkholder, W.J., & Toll, P.W. 2000. Obesity. In M.S. Hand, C.D. Thatcher, R.L. Remillard, & P. Roudebush (eds.), *Small animal clinical nutrition* (4th. ed., pp. 405–406). Marceline, MO: Walsworth Publishing for Mark Morris Institute.

Burkholder, W.J. 2000. Precision and practicality of methods assessing body composition of dogs and cats. In *Nutrition forum proceedings* (pp. 1-9). St. Louis, MO: Ralston Purina Co.

Case, L.P., Carey, D.P., Hirakawa, D.A., & Daristotle, L. 2000. Adult maintenance. In *Canine and feline nutrition: A resource for companion animal professionals* (2nd. ed., pp. 256–257). St. Louis, MO: Mosby.

19

Pregnancy and Lactation in Dogs

Nutrition for the bitch during gestation and lactation should take place long before she is bred or the litter is whelped. Before breeding, both the sire and the dam should be in excellent physical condition, moderate body condition, and well exercised. They should both have complete physical examinations by a veterinarian; be current on all preventative health programs such as vaccinations, heartworm medications, and intestinal dewormers; and be tested for the presence of brucellosis and herpes virus (Buffington et al., 2004; Case et al., 2000). If this is a pure-bred litter, both parents should also be screened for any congenital problems, as well as shown to adhere to established breed standards (Case et al., 2000).

If the bitch is underweight, she may not be able to consume enough food during the pregnancy to provide for both her physical needs and the needs of her developing puppies. Lack of proper nutrition in the bitch can result in decreased birth weight and increased neonatal mortality (Case et al., 2000). A bitch that is overweight at the time of breeding may be predisposed to the development of very large puppies and resultant dystocia, which puts the life of both the bitch and puppies at risk. Obesity has also been shown to decrease ovulation rates, produce smaller litters, and provide insufficient milk production after gestation (Debraekeleer et al., 2000). It is recommended that overweight bitches lose weight before breeding to optimize fertility and decrease the risk of developing dystocia (Debraekeleer et al., 2000).

What to Feed

If the breeding pair is in good physical and nutritional condition, no special foods need to be fed before or during the breeding. Feeding a complete and balanced, highly digestible diet that has undergone feeding trials for pregnancy and lactation is recommended (Buffinton et al., 2004; Case et al., 2000; Debraekeleer et al., 2000). It is not unusual for the bitch to have a slightly depressed appetite during estrus; this can be due to hormonal changes as well as nervousness (Case et al., 2000; Debraekeleer et al., 2000). The diet should be changed if needed early in her reproductive cycle to allow her to fully adjust to the new food before breeding and to help prevent any abrupt change in diet during gestation or lactation (Case et al., 2000).

Gestation is a unique situation in which nutritional requirements increase markedly over a relatively short period of time (Debraekeleer et al., 2000). It is suggested to increase the amount of food fed to the bitch by 15% each week from the fifth week of gestation until parturition. Following this regimen would mean that by whelping, the bitch will be eating 60% more food than when she was mated (LeGrand-Defretin & Munday, 1995). As the pregnancy advances, it is reasonable to decrease the size of the meals and offer them more frequently. This allows a bitch with a large litter and little free abdominal space to still meet her energy requirements (LeGrand-Defretin & Munday, 1995).

The Puppies

Although the puppies are developing rapidly, they are very small until the last third of the 63-day gestation (Case et al., 2000). They have little impact on the bitch's weight and nutritional needs until after the fifth week of pregnancy. After the fifth week, fetal size and weight increase rapidly for the remaining 3 to 4 weeks of gestation. In the dog, greater than 75% of the weight and at least half of the fetal length are attained between the 40th and 55th days of gestation (Case et al., 2000).

Lactation

Lactation presents the greatest test of nutritional adequacy of any feeding regimen (LeGrand-Defretin & Munday, 1995). The bitch must eat, digest, absorb, and use large amounts of nutrients to produce sufficient milk of adequate quality to support the growth and development of several puppies (LeGrand-Defretin & Munday, 1995). Not only does she need to meet the entire energy requirements for the rapidly growing puppies, but also she must be able to meet all of her energy and nutrient requirements. The amount of energy needed to meet these multiple requirements is dependent on the normal energy intake of the bitch and the size and age of the litter (LeGrand-Defretin & Munday, 1995). A 5 lb. Maltese with two puppies would require much less energy per pound than would a 15 lb. Beagle with six puppies (LeGrand-Defretin & Munday, 1995). The bitch does not require additional vitamin or mineral supplements if a balanced diet suitable for gestation and lactation is being fed (LeGrand-Defretin & Munday, 1995).

After whelping, the bitch's energy requirement steadily increases and peaks between 3 and 5 weeks postpartum to a level two to four times higher than daily energy requirements (DER) for nonlactating adults (Debraekeleer et al., 2000). The energy requirements return to normal levels about 8 weeks postpartum (Debraekeleer et al., 2000). If the energy density of the food is too low, the bitch may not be able to physically consume enough food to meet both her and the puppies' energy requirements. If this happens, her milk production will decrease, she will lose weight, and she may display signs of severe exhaustion (Debraekeleer et al., 2000). This is most pronounced in giant-breed dogs with large litters (Debraekeleer et al., 2000).

Water is of utmost importance during lactation. Inadequate water intake leads to a significant decrease in the quantity of milk produced. Fresh, cool water should always be readily available to the lactating bitch (Case et al., 2000).

As a rough estimate, a lactating bitch would require 1.9 $\times$ resting energy requirement (RER) plus 25% of this amount for each puppy.

TABLE 19.1. **Example.**

60 lb. Labrador (prepregnancy weight) with 7 puppies

60 lb. = 27.3 kg

RER = (30 $\times$ wt [in kg]) + 70

RER = (30 $\times$ 27.3 kg) + 70 = 889

Lactation = RER $\times$ 1.9 = 1,689 kcal/day

25% for each puppy = 422.25 kcal/puppy

7 puppies = 2,955.75 kcal/day

Bitch + puppies = 1,689 + 2,955.75 = 4,644.75 kcal/day

Commercial dry puppy food = 375 kcal/cup

Feed 12.4 cups/day

References

Buffington, T., Holloway, C.A., & Abood, S.K. 2004. Normal dogs. In *Manual of veterinary dietetics* (pp. 9–11). St. Louis, MO: Elsevier.

Case, L.P., Carey, D.P., Hirakawa, D.A., & Daristotle, L. 2000. Pregnancy and lactation. In *Canine and feline nutrition: A resource for companion animal professionals* (2nd. ed., pp. 225–232). St. Louis, MO: Mosby.

Debraekeleer, J., Gross, K.L., & Zicker, S.C. 2000. Normal dogs. In M.S. Hand, C.D. Thatcher, R.L. Remillard, & P. Roudebush (eds.), *Small animal clinical nutrition* (4th. ed., pp. 232–241). Marceline, MO: Walsworth Publishing for Mark Morris Institute.

LeGrand-Defretin, V., & Munday, H.S. 1995. Feeding dogs and cats for life. In I.H. Burger (ed.), *The Waltham book of companion animal nutrition* (pp. 57–59). Oxford: Butterworth-Heinemann.

20

Pregnancy and Lactation in Cats

As with dogs, any cat being considered for breeding should be in excellent physical condition, moderate body condition, and well exercised. Both the queen and tom should have complete physical examinations by a veterinarian; be current on all preventative health programs such as vaccinations, heartworm medications, and intestinal dewormers; and be tested for the presence of feline leukemia virus and feline immunodeficiency virus (Buffington et al., 2004; Case et al., 2000). If this is a pure-bred litter, both parents should also be screened for any congenital problems as well as shown to adhere to established breed standards (Case et al., 2000).

Domestic cats generally have their first heat cycles between 6 to 9 months of age. This does not mean that they are physically ready to have a litter of kittens. Before 10 to 12 months of age, queens are still growing, and if they become pregnant must support not only their own continued growth but also that of their kittens (Kirk et al., 2000). The best age for breeding is between $1^1/_2$ and 7 years of age. Queens older than 7 years should not be bred due to reproductive complications, irregular estrous cycles, and reduced litter size (Kirk et al., 2000).

Queens that are underweight or in poor body condition may fail to conceive, abort, or bear small underweight kittens. They may also have markedly reduced lactation. Obesity in cats can lead to large kittens, resulting in increased incidence of dystocia (Kirk et al., 2000).

What to Feed

Unlike most species, weight gain in a queen increases linearly from conception to parturition. This weight gain in early pregnancy is not associated with significant growth of reproductive tissues or fetal growth but appears to be stored in energy deposits (presumably as fat) to support lactation (Case et al., 2000; Kirk et al., 2000). This stored energy can account for up to 60% of the weight gained during the pregnancy and is gradually lost during lactation (Case et al., 2000). The average weight gain should be about 40% of the premating weight (Kirk et al., 2000).

The queen should be fed a diet that is intended for reproduction throughout gestation and lactation (Case et al., 2000; Kirk et al., 2000). The amount of food should be gradually increased, beginning at the second week of gestation and continuing until parturition. At the end of gestation, the queen should be consuming about 25% to 50% more food than during her normal maintenance needs (Case et al., 2000).

The Kittens

Kittens should exhibit steady weight gain, have good muscle tone, and suckle vigorously. Young kittens are quiet between feedings (Kirk et al., 2000). Kittens that are restless and cry excessively may not be receiving enough milk due to poor lactation. Gastric distention is not a good indicator of adequate nursing. Excessive swallowing of air during nursing can give the appearance of gastric fullness, despite inadequate milk intake (Kirk et al., 2000). Kitten mortality reportedly varies from 9% to 63% depending on the source of the cats and the cattery (Kirk et al., 2000). Several genetic, husbandry, and nutritional factors can contribute to high mortality. If kitten death or cannibalism by the queen is high, all three areas should be investigated (Kirk et al., 2000).

Lactation

Lactation presents the biggest test of nutritional adequacy of any feeding regimen (LeGrand–Defretin & Munday, 1995). The queen must eat, digest, absorb, and use large amounts of nutrients to produce sufficient milk of adequate quality to support the growth and development of several kittens (LeGrand–Defretin & Munday, 1995). Not only does she need to meet the entire energy requirements for the rapidly growing kittens, but also she must be able to meet all of her energy and nutrient requirements. The amount of energy needed to meet these multiple requirements is dependent on the normal energy intake of the queen and the size and age of the litter (LeGrand–Defretin & Munday, 1995).

Depending on litter size, the queen should be eating two to three times her maintenance energy requirements (MER) during lactation (Case et al., 2000). A general guideline is to feed 1.5 x MER during the first week of lactation, 2 x MER during the second week, and 2.5 to 3 ×MER during the fourth week of lactation (Case et al., 2000). If the energy density of the food is too low, the queen may not be able to physically consume enough food to meet both her and the kittens' energy requirements. If this happens, her milk production will decrease, she will lose weight, and she may display signs of severe exhaustion (Kirk et al., 2000).

Milk production depends on litter size and stage of lactation (Kirk et al., 2000). Peak lactation occurs between 3 and 4 weeks postpartum (Kirk et al., 2000). Continuous weight gain by the kitten is the best indicator of adequate milk production by the queen (Kirk et al., 2000).

Water is of utmost importance during lactation. Inadequate water intake heads to a significant decrease in the quantity of milk produced. Fresh, cool water should always be readily available to the lactating queen (Case et al., 2000).

References

Buffington, T., Holloway, C.A., & Abood, S.K. 2004. Nornal cats. In *Manual of veterinary dietetics* (pp. 27–38). St. Louis, MO: Elsevier.

Case, L.P., Carey, D.P., Hirakawa, D.A., & Daristotle, L. 2000. Pregnancy and lactation. In *Canine and feline nutrition: A resource for companion animal professionals* (2nd. ed., pp. 225–232). St. Louis, MO: Mosby.

Kirk, C.L., Debraekeleer, J., & Armstrong, P.J. 2000. Normal cats. In M.S. Hand, C.D. Thatcher, R.L. Remillard, & P. Roudebush (eds.), *Small animal clinical nutrition* (4th. ed., pp. 320–328). Marceline, MO: Walsworth Publishing for Mark Morris Institute.

LeGrand–Defretin, V., & Munday, H.S. 1995. Feeding dogs and cats for life. In I.H. Burger (ed.), *The Waltham book of companion animal nutrition* (pp. 57–59). Oxford: Butterworth–Heinemann.

21

Neonatal Puppies and Kittens

The first week of a newborn's life is the most critical for its survival. Newborn puppies and kittens are physiologically immature, with low percentages of body fat—1% to 2% compared with 12% to 35% in adults. They do not develop adequate glycogen reserves until after the first few days of nursing (Buffington et al., 2004).

Nutrition

The first nutritional concern for newborns is that they receive colostrum immediately after birth. Colostrum is milk produced by the mother during the first 24 to 72 hours after parturition. Colostrum provides nutrients, water, growth factors, digestive enzymes, and maternal immunoglobulins (antibodies) (Kirk et al., 2000). All of these are critical to the survival of the newborn. The main difference between colostrum and milk is in the water content and nutrient composition (Kirk et al., 2000). The water content of colostrum is lower than that of milk, which accounts for its sticky, concentrated appearance compared with regular milk. The water content found in the milk will gradually increase from day 1 to day 3 (Kirk et al., 2000). Lactose concentrations found in colostrum are also lower than those found in milk, with protein and fat levels being higher. Energy content in milk also increases throughout lactation (Kirk et al., 2000).

Maintenance of body temperature is the second most important concern for newborns. Neonatal puppies and kittens are unable to thermoregulate and must be kept in an environment that is 85 to 90°F during the first week of life and 80 to 85°F during the second week (Buffington et al., 2004). If the neonates are not kept warm enough and develop hypothermia, they will be unable to eat, and if tube fed, they will be unable to digest the food. This failure to eat may result in rejection by the bitch or queen (Buffington et al., 2004). The best source of warmth is the mother. After 6 days, the neonates are able to shiver but are still very susceptible to chilling. Keeping the environment warm and free of drafts is of utmost importance during the first few weeks of life (Case et al., 2000).

Motherless neonates have the same requirements as do neonates that have a mother—they still need adequate nutrition and warmth. Obviously, the best course for the young puppy or kitten would be to have a foster mother; if this is not available, they can be hand-reared. If they are hand-reared, not only do they need to be fed, but they also have to have their urination and defecation stimulated. This will need to be continued until the puppies or kittens are between 16 and 21 days old (Debraekeleer et al., 2000).

Milk from other species is an inadequate substitute for mother's milk. The protein, fat, and calcium levels found in goat and cow milk are too low for either puppies or kittens (Debraekeleer et al., 2000). Queen's milk would also be inadequate for puppies because of lactose and calcium levels. Bitch's milk contains almost twice as much protein as cow milk. It also provides branched chain amino acids and high levels of arginine and lysine (Debraekeleer et al., 2000).

TABLE 21.1. **Nutrient composition of various milks.**

Nutrient	Queen's Milk	Bitch's Milk	Cow Milk	Goat Milk
Moisture (g/100 g)	79	77.3	87.7	87.0
Crude protein (g/100 g)	7.5	7.5	3.3	3.6
Crude fat (g/100 g)	8.5	9.5	3.6	4.1
Lactose (g/100 g)	4.0	3.3	4.7	4.0
Calcium (mg/100 g)	180	240	119	133
ME (kcal/100 g)	121	146	64	69

From Kirk, C.L., Debraekeleer, J., & Armstrong, P.J. 2000. Normal cats. In M.S. Hand, C.D. Thatcher, R.L. Remillard, & P. Roudebush (eds.), *Small animal clinical nutrition* (4th. ed., pp. 331–332). Marceline, MO: Walsworth Publishing for Mark Morris Institute.

Surveys indicate that a high percentage of deaths before weaning are due to a relatively small number of causes—infectious diseases, congenital defects, and malnutrition (Buffington et al., 2004). The cause of malnutrition is usually from death of or neglect from the mother, lactation failure, or a litter that is too large for the milk supply (Buffington et al., 2004).

If the puppies or kittens are raised by their mother, they should be allowed free access to her. The puppies or kittens should be monitored to ensure that they are receiving adequate nutrition and have received colostrum during the first 24 hours of life (Debraekeleer et al., 2000). During the first few weeks of life, they should nurse at least four to six times per day. In healthy puppies and kittens, the mother's milk supports normal growth until approximately 4 weeks of age (Case et al., 2000). Supplemental feedings should be necessary only with unusually large litters or with maternal rejection (Case et al., 2000). After 4 weeks of age, milk alone does not provide adequate calories or nutrients for continued normal development (Case et al., 2000).

Milk Replacers

Commercially available milk replacers can be used to supply or supplement the nutritional needs of neonates. Most milk replacers are based on cow or goat milk and modified to more resemble the nutrient profile for bitch's and queen's milk (LeGrand-Defretin & Munday, 1995).

While there are "home-made" recipes for milk replacers for puppies and kittens, most of these recipes were developed through trial and error, and their actual nutrient content is unknown (Case et al., 2000). If fed straight cow milk, neonate puppies develop severe diarrhea. Cow milk contains nearly three times the lactose found in bitch's milk (Case et al., 2000). Cow milk also contains an excessive proportion of casein for neonatal puppies and kittens and supplies insufficient calories for both (Case et al., 2000).

Commercial milk replacers are the preferred source of nutrition for orphans or as supplemental feeding (Case et al., 2000). A product that has been tested for the specific purpose of raising neonatal puppies or kittens should be selected. Even though the nutrient content and bioavailability are guaranteed, commercial formulas vary in their ability to provide adequate nutrition and calories (Case et al., 2000).

The Association of American Feed Control Officials (AAFCO) does not provide detailed guidelines for testing milk replacers. It is important to obtain manufacturer's information related to nutrient composition, nutritional integrity, and feeding efficacy (Case et al., 2000). It is important to remember that even the best milk replacer can not provide the neonate with the antibodies found in colostrum; therefore, extra care must be taken to maintain a clean environment and prevent transmission of disease (Case et al., 2000).

Weaning

Weaning is a gradual process with two phases. The first phase begins when the neonate begins to eat solid food between 3 and 4 weeks of age (Case et al., 2000; Kirk et al., 2000). This can be encouraged by mixing a commercial food specifically made for weaning puppies and kittens or by making a thick gruel by mixing a small amount of warm water with the mother's food. This semisolid food should be provided in a shallow dish, with the puppies or kittens allowed free access to the fresh food several times per day (Case et al., 2000; Kirk et al., 2000). The food should be removed after 20 to 30 minutes to discourage bacterial growth in the food.

Initially, the intake of food will be minimal, but by 5 to 6 weeks of age, the deciduous teeth will have begun to erupt, enabling the puppies and kittens to chew and eat dry food (Case et al., 2000; Kirk et al., 2000). As the food intake increases in the neonates, the mother's milk production will decrease. By 6 weeks of age, the second stage of weaning can begin with the puppies and kittens obtaining their full nutrition from their food and not from their mother (nutritional weaning) (Case et al., 2000; Kirk et al., 2000). Even though some mothers will continue to nurse their young past this time, very little milk is being produced with little nutrition being obtained. It is believed that the psychological and emotional benefits of suckling may be as important as the nutritional benefits in animals that are older than 5 weeks (Case et al., 2000). For this reason, complete weaning (behavioral weaning) should not be done until puppies and kittens are at least 7 to 8 weeks of age (Case et al., 2000).

References

Buffington, T., Holloway, C.A., & Abood, S.K. 2004. Nornal dogs. In *Manual of veterinary dietetics* (pp. 11–12). St. Louis, MO: Elsevier.
Case, L.P., Carey, D.P., Hirakawa, D.A., & Daristotle, L. 2000. Nutritional care of neonatal puppies and kittens. In *Canine and feline nutrition: A resource for companion animal professionals* (2nd. ed., pp. 233–243). St. Louis, MO: Mosby.

Debraekeleer, J., Gross, K.L., & Zicker, S.C. 2000. Normal dogs. In M.S. Hand, C.D. Thatcher, R.L. Remillard, & P. Roudebush (eds.), *Small animal clinical nutrition* (4th. ed., pp. 244–247). Marceline, MO: Walsworth Publishing for Mark Morris Institute.

Kirk, C.L., Debraekeleer, J., & Armstrong, P.J. 2000. Normal cats. In M.S. Hand, C.D. Thatcher, R.L. Remillard, & P. Roudebush (eds.), *Small animal clinical nutrition* (4th. ed., pp. 331–332). Marceline, MO: Walsworth Publishing for Mark Morris Institute.

LeGrand-Defretin, V., & Munday, H.S. 1995. Feeding dogs and cats for life. In I.H. Burger (ed.), *The Waltham book of companion animal nutrition* (pp. 61–65). Oxford: Butterworth-Heinemann.

22

Growth in Dogs

The dog is unique among other mammals in that it has the widest range of normal adult body weight within any single species, ranging in size from adult Yorkshire Terriers and Chihuahuas weighing only 3 lb. to adult Great Danes and Mastiffs that can top 200 lb. (LeGrand-Defretin & Munday, 1995). Because of this wide range in sizes, growth in the early stages of life is very rapid and, in general, most breeds of dog will reach 50% of their adult weight at between 5 and 6 months old (LeGrand-Defretin & Munday, 1995). Different breeds will continue to mature at different rates, with some of the larger breeds not reaching maturity until almost 2 years of age.

After nursing, postweaning growth is the most nutritionally demanding period in a dog's life. With large- and giant-breed dogs, the length and speed of their growth pose an even higher nutritional demand. First, we address normal growth, and then we see how this differs with the large and giant breeds. Obviously what works nutritionally for a Chihuahua will not necessarily work for an Irish Wolfhound.

Normal Growth

The most rapid period of growth is seen during the first 6 months of life. With this comes the increased requirement for all nutrients, with energy and calcium being of special concern (Gross et al., 2000). Most small-breed dogs will have reached their adult size by 8 to 12 months, medium-breed dogs by 12 to 18 months, and large- and giant-breed dogs not until 18 to 24 months (Case et al., 2000). By maturity, most dogs will have increased their birth weight by 40 to 50 times (Case et al., 2000).

Diet restriction, and thus energy restriction, has been shown to affect the life span of dogs, with the primary research being done on Labrador Retrievers over the span of 15 years. All dogs were housed in the same conditions, received the same level of care, and were fed the same food; the only difference between the two groups was in the amount of food consumed. One group of 24 dogs was designated the control group and was fed 62.1 kcal of ME/kg of estimated ideal body weight; the remaining 24 dogs were fed 25% less than their pairmate. The group fed the larger amount had a body condition score of 6/9 to 7/9, with the restricted group having body condition scores of 4/9 to 5/9, with a score of 1 being emaciated and a score of 9 being severely obese. The group that received the larger amount of food on average died 2 years earlier than their pairmates, developed osteoarthritis 1.1 years sooner, and developed chronic health conditions 6 months sooner (Kealy et al., 2002). The only difference between these two groups was the amount of food fed. Following body condition scoring, none of the group fed the larger amounts were obese, and none of the restricted fed dogs were emaciated; these were all "average" sized Labradors.

This group of Labradors were fed controlled amounts from the time they entered the study at 6 weeks of age until they either died or were euthanized (Kealy et al., 2002). Because of the rapid growth that is seen in dogs during the first 12 to 18 months, this restriction can become very important when we are looking at the development of orthopedic problems later in life. While these problems occur later in life, they do not develop later in life but rather while the dog is going through this rapid growth phase.

Even though calcium is essential for bone growth, the actual requirements in puppies are quite low. The Association of American Feed Control Officials (AAFCO)'s Nutrient Profiles recommend that dog foods formulated for growth contain a minimum of 1% calcium on a dry-matter basis (Case et al., 2000). In general, calcium absorption from the food is dependent on requirements and calcium intake (Gross et al., 2000).

What to Feed

The protein requirements for growing puppies are higher than that for adult dogs, because not only does the puppy have normal maintenance needs but also it needs protein to build new tissue associated with growth (Case et al., 2000). Because puppies eat higher amounts of energy, the total amount of protein eaten is naturally higher. Foods fed to growing puppies should contain slightly higher levels of protein than those fed for adult maintenance. Most important, this protein should be of high quality and highly digestible (Case et al., 2000). The minimum level of protein found in puppy diets should be 22% of the ME, with optimal levels between 25% and 29%. The type of protein included in the diet should be of high quality to ensure that all of the essential amino acids are being delivered to the body for use in growth and development (Case et al., 2000).

Because of the quantity of food needed to meet energy requirements, energy density is very important for growing puppies. If they are fed a poor quality diet with low energy density and low digestibility, they need to consume large quantities to meet their energy requirements (Gross et al., 2000). This intake of large volumes of food can increase the incidence of flatulence, vomiting, and diarrhea and the development of a "pot-bellied" appearance (Gross et al., 2000).

While puppies do have increased requirements for energy and other essential nutrients compared with adults, they also tend to have less digestive capacity, smaller mouths, and smaller and fewer teeth with which to eat their food. This is especially true for small and toy breeds of dogs (Case et al., 2000). These differences limit the amount of food that the puppy can consume and digest within a meal or a given amount of time (Case et al., 2000).

It is equally important to not overfeed growing dogs; not only can this lead to an accelerated growth rate, but also causes buildup of adipose tissue that can contribute to obesity later in life (Case et al., 2000). Many well-meaning owners supplement an otherwise balanced diet, causing nutrient excessive that would not have existed before. It is not advised to supplement a balanced diet—if the owner feels that a supplement is needed, maybe the diet should be changed instead to a better-quality diet.

Feeding Regimens

When a new puppy is initially brought home, the diet should not be changed from what had been fed previously, unless the food was of a very poor quality. Moving to a new home and leaving the bitch and littermates is quite stressful for a young dog (Case et al., 2000). A new diet can be introduced 2 to 3 days after the move home, although it is best to do this transition slowly over 5 to 7 days. The easiest way to do this is to mix the food in quarters—on day 1, give ³/₄ of the old diet mixed with ¹/₄ of the new diet; on days 2 and 3, give ½ of the old diet mixed with ½ of the new diet' on days 4 and 5, give ¼ of the old diet with ¾ of the new diet; and on day 6, the transition is complete (Gross et al., 2000).

Free-choice and time-restricted feedings are not recommended for puppies. Free-choice feedings may increase the amount of body fat, predisposing the dog to obesity later in life and cause skeletal deformities at a young age. Studies using time-restricted feedings have shown that the puppies increase body weight, have more body fat, and increase bone mineralization faster than puppies fed free-choice (Gross et al., 2000). During periods of rapid growth, it is better to do measured feedings two to four times per day. The amount fed should be based on the growth rate of the dog and the BCS. The feeding guides listed on the package can be used as a starting point. Puppies should be lean, not skinny nor not roly-poly, throughout their growth phase.

Large- and Giant-Breed Puppies

Nutrient excesses, rapid growth rates, and excessive weight gain appear to be important factors contributing to the incidence of skeletal disorders in growing large- and giant-breed dogs (Kuhlman & Biourge, 1997). While we continue to select for increased size for many of our larger dogs, size itself is not detrimental to the dog, but management practices that allow growth rate to be maximized can cause the negative consequences that we see in these dogs (Lepine & Reinhart, 1998).

It is well documented that the incidence of skeletal disease, including osteochoncrosis (OCD), hypertrophic osteodystrophy, and hip dysplasia (CHD), is markedly increased in the growing large-breed dog if management practices are such that this maximal genetic potential for rate of growth is realized (Lepine & Reinhart, 1998). The primary management practice affecting growth rate and ultimately skeletal disease is nutritional support (Lepine & Reinhart, 1998).

The primary nutritional considerations implicated in skeletal disease development in growing large-breed dogs are dietary concentrations of protein, energy, and calcium (Lepine & Reinhart, 1998).

Hip Dysplasia

CHD is a disease of dogs in which abnormal development of the hip joint results due to disparity between the strength of the soft tissues supporting the joint and the increasing biomechanical forces associated with weight gain. This causes the coxofemoral joint to not "fit" properly; this subluxation causes remodeling of the joint including a shallowing of the acetabulum, a flattening of the femoral head, and eventually osteoarthritis (Kuhlman & Biourge, 1997; Lepine & Reinhart, 1998). CHD can affect any breed but is more prevalent in large-breed dogs, and is generally accepted as polygenic in its inheritance (Kuhlman & Biourge, 1997; Lepine & Reinhart, 1998). This means that the disease is not caused by one gene but by a combination of multiple genes and outside factors.

A controlled study conducted on Labrador Retrievers showed that significantly less hip joint laxity and a lower incidence of CHD were seen in the group of dogs receiving 25% less food than their pairmates. The food-restricted group grew at a slower rate than those receiving 25% more food; this is believed to be the reason for the significant decrease in CHD (Kealy et al., 2002; Kuhlman & Biourge, 1997). In the food-restricted group, 16 of 24 developed osteoarthiritis, with the mean age of onset 13.3 years; for the unrestricted group, 19 of 24 dogs developed osteoarthritis, with the mean age of onset 10.3 years (Kealy et al., 2002).

Osteochondrosis

OCD is a focal area of disruption in the endochondral ossification and is characterized by impaired maturation of chondrocytes and delayed cartilage mineralization (Kuhlman & Biourge, 1997; Richardson, 1999). The most commonly affected joints are the shoulder, elbow, hock, and stifle. Acute pain and swelling are seen in the affected areas, and stiffness and lameness aggravated by exercise often result (Kuhlman & Biourge, 1997). It is believed that overnutrition as the result of ad-lib feeding stimulates skeletal growth, bone remodeling, and weight gain in breeds already having a genetic potential for rapid growth (Richardson, 1999). This combination of rapid growth and remodeling weakens the subchondral region in its support of the cartilage surface (Richardson, 1999). The increasing body weight exerts excessive biomechanical forces on the cartilage and leads to secondary disturbances in chondrocyte nutrition, metabolism, function, and viability (Richardson, 1999). Acute inflammatory joint disease begins when the subchondral bone is exposed to synovial fluid. Inflammatory mediators and cartilage fragments are released into the joint and perpetuate the cycle of degenerative joint disease (Richardson, 1999). In a rapidly growing puppy, overnutrition can result in a mismatch between body weight and skeletal growth, which can lead to overloading of the skeletal structures (Richardson, 1999).

What to Feed

Overnutrition to achieve maximal growth rate causes excessive body weight, which overloads the young skeleton and may contribute to the development of skeletal disorders (Kuhlman & Biourge, 1997). Because fats contain more than twice the caloric density of protein and carbohydrates, a diet lower in fat is recommended for large- and giant-breed puppies (Kuhlman & Biourge, 1997).

A BCS of 2/5 to 3/5, or 4/9, should be maintained throughout puppyhood (Richardson, 1999). Limiting energy intake to maintain these physical parameters will not affect the dog's progress toward its ultimate genetic potential, but it will reduce food intake, fecal output, obesity, and the risk of skeletal disease (Richardson, 1999).

Protein has not been shown to have any negative consequences on calcium metabolism or skeletal development in the dog (Richardson, 1999). A minimum level of protein in the diet depends on digestibility, amino acid profile, and bioavailability (Richardson, 1999).

The absolute level of calcium rather than a calcium—phosphorus imbalance is responsible for negatively influencing skeletal development (Richardson, 1999). Young large-breed dogs fed a diet high in calcium have a significant increase in incidence of developmental skeletal disease (Richardson, 1999). Large-breed puppies should not be switched to an adult maintenance diet too early, because of the difference in energy density between a puppy diet and an adult diet; the puppy would actually consume more calcium in an adult diet because it would need to eat more to meet its energy needs (Richardson, 1999). Under no circumstances should these puppies receive calcium supplements (Richardson, 1999).

Feeding Regimens

A combination of time-restricted and measured feedings are recommended for large- and giant-breed puppies (Richardson, 1999). Because of their steep growth curve, measured feedings may not be able to keep up with their energy requirements, and frequent body weight checks and caloric recalculations would be necessary to provide the proper amount of food. When combined with time-restricted feedings offered two to three times a day, enough energy can be provided for growth but not too much, as would be seen with ad-lib feeding (Richardson, 1999). Frequent assessment of BCS will help to determine the proper amount of food to offer the puppy.

If puppies are fed based on energy requirements, activity levels, and body condition, growth diets do not increase the risk of developmental bone disease in large- and giant-breed dogs (Richardson, 1999). It is important not only to feed the appropriate diet but also to feed the diet appropriately! (Richardson, 1999).

TABLE 22.1. **Nutrient profiles.**

SMALL BREED PUPPY FOOD DRY

Caloric Distribution (% ME)

Protein: 29%
Fat: 46%
Carbohydrate: 25%
Calories: 485 kcal/cup

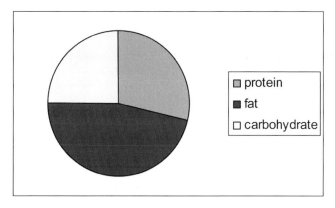

LARGE BREED PUPPY FOOD DRY

Caloric Distribution (% ME)

Protein: 25%
Fat: 36%
Carbohydrate: 39%
Calories: 362 kcal/cup

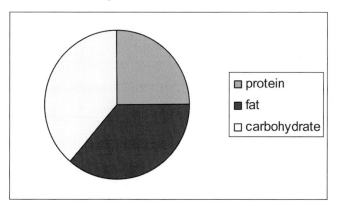

(Continued)

TABLE 22.1.   (*Continued*)

ADULT MAINTENANCE FOOD DRY

Caloric distribution (% ME)

Protein: 24%
Fat: 38%
Carbohydrate: 38%
Calories: 405 kcal/cup

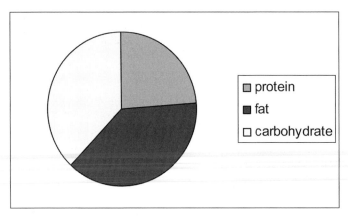

ADULT MAINTENANCE LARGE BREED DRY

Caloric Distribution (% ME)

Protein: 24%
Fat: 33%
Carbohydrate: 43%
Calories: 344 kcal/cup

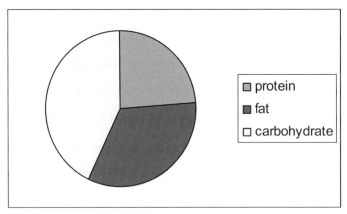

From Eukanuba. 2003. *Veterinary diets product reference guide* (pp. 69-71). Dayton, OH: Iams Co.

References

Case, L.P., Carey, D.P., Hirakawa, D.A., & Daristotle, L. 2000. Growth. In *Canine and feline nutrition: A resource for companion animal professionals* (2nd. ed., pp. 245–254). St. Louis, MO: Mosby.

Gross, K.L., Wedekind, K.L., Cowell, C.S., Schoenherr,, W.D., Jewell, D.E., Zicker, S.C., Debraekeleer, J., & Frey, R.A. 2000. Normal dogs. In M.S. Hand, C.D. Thatcher, R.L. Remillard, & P. Roudebush (eds.), *Small animal clinical nutrition* (4th. ed., pp. 247–250). Marceline, MO: Walsworth Publishing for Mark Morris Institute.

Kealy, R.D., Lawler, D.F., Ballam, J.M., Mantz, S.L., Biery, D.N., Greeley, E.H., Lust, G., Segre, M., Smith, G.K., & Stowe, H.D. 2002. Effects of diet restriction on life span and age-related changes in dogs. In *Journal of the American Veterinary Medical Association, 220,* 1315–1320.

Kuhlman, G., & Biourge, V. 1997. Nutrition of the large and giant breed dog with emphasis on skeletal development. *Veterinary Clinical Nutrition, 4,* 89–95.

LeGrand-Defretin, V., & Munday, H.S. 1995. Feeding dogs and cats for life. In I.H. Burger (ed.), *The Waltham book of companion animal nutrition* (pp. 63–64). Oxford: Butterworth-Heinemann.

Lepine, A.J., & Reinhart, G.A. 1998. Feeding the growing large breed dog. In *Clinical Nutrition Symposium XXIII Congress of the World Small Animal Veterinary Association* (pp. 12–16). Buenos Aires, October 6, 1998. Dayton, OH: Iams Co.

Richardson, D.C. 2000. Developmental orthopedics: Nutritional influences in the dog. In S.J. Ettinger & E.C. Feldman (eds.), *Textbook of veterinary internal medicine: Diseases of the dog and cat* (5th. ed., pp. 252–258). Philadelphia: W.B. Saunders.

23

Growth in Cats

Unlike dogs, cats do not have a wide variety of sizes or shapes, and they do not have as rapid of a growth phase. But like dogs, they should be fed to achieve normal growth and development (Case et al., 2000).

Normal Growth

As young animals, kittens have a small physical capacity for food, so it is not only recommended to feed energy-dense foods but to feed them frequently (LeGrand-Defretin & Munday, 1995). The ultimate goal of feeding kittens is to ensure a healthy adult cat. The objective is to optimize growth, minimize risk factors for disease, and achieve optimal health (Kirk et al., 2000). Energy requirements are highest at about 10 weeks of age; after this point, the energy requirements per unit of body weight gradually decrease, although they remain relatively high for at least the first 6 months of life (LeGrand-Defretin & Munday, 1995). Most cats will achieve skeletal maturity at about 10 months of age, even though not all growth plates may have closed by this time (Kirk et al., 2000). Additional weight gain may occur after 12 months of age and represents a phase of maturation and muscle development (Kirk et al., 2000).

Growing kittens have high energy requirements to meet the needs of rapid growth, thermoregulation, and maintenance needs (Kirk et al., 2000). Feeding an energy-dense food allows for smaller volumes to be consumed to satisfy caloric needs (Kirk et al., 2000). However, cats with BCS of 4/5 or 6/9 should be fed foods with less energy density to prevent obesity. The prevalence of obesity increase after 1 year of age, and overnutrition is more of a problem in most kittens than undernutrition (Kirk et al., 2000).

There is no evidence that the age of neutering alters the rate of growth. Unfortunately, energy requirements do decline with neutering, increasing the risk of obesity if energy intake is not adjusted (Kirk et al., 2000). Obesity should be prevented in young cats as this increases the number of fat cells capable of storing fat as the cat enters adulthood. Neutering reduces energy requirements by 24% to 33% regardless of the age at neutering (Kirk et al., 2000).

What to Feed

The requirement for protein is already relatively high for the adult cat; it is even higher for growth kittens by about 10% (LeGrand-Defretin & Munday, 1995). At least 19% of the protein should be from an animal source to ensure adequate amounts of the sulfur-containing amino acids, which are required in larger amounts in kittens than in other species (Kirk et al., 2000). Taurine, one of the sulfur-containing amino acids, has a well-documented role in reproduction and growth, and all foods for growing kittens should contain adequate amounts (Kirk et al., 2000). The Association of American Feed Control Officials (AAFCO) recommends a minimum protein level of 26% ME (Kirk et al., 2000).

The palatability of the food should be good enough to ensure adequate energy intake, with a digestibility of at least 80% and protein digestibility of at least 85% (Kirk et al., 2000).

Carbohydrates are not required in the food used for growing kittens as long as sufficient gluconeogenic amino acids are available (Kirk et al., 2000). Cats can readily digest carbohydrates, although feeding a diet high in poorly digestible carbohydrates may result in flatulence, bloating, and diarrhea (Kirk et al., 2000). This can often be seen in kittens fed cow milk after weaning. Cow milk has higher levels of lactose than does cat milk and, after weaning, a kitten's level of lactase, the enzyme that breaks down lactose, declines (Kirk et al., 2000).

A high-quality commercial kitten food that has been shown to be adequate for growth through AAFCO feeding trials is recommended (Case et al., 2000). Supplementation of this diet is not recommended and should not be necessary (Case et al., 2000).

It is better to change to a food specifically formulated for kittens than to try to balance an inappropriate food (Kirk et al., 2000). A balanced kitten food can be fed until kittens reach adulthood at approximately 10 to 12 months of age (Kirk et al., 2000). If a kitten is showing signs of obesity, it can be switched to a balanced adult diet by 6 months of age (LeGrand-Defretin & Munday, 1995).

Feeding Regimens

Free-choice feeding is often preferred with kittens because it reduces the risk of underfeeding and reduces the marked gastric distention that sometimes accompanies rapid meal feeding in kittens (Kirk et al., 2000). This feeding method may not be a good option if older cats are in the house, as they may push the kitten away from the food and eat it all themselves. Measured feedings can be used in a mixed age household if two or three meals per day are offered and everyone is fed in separate areas to allow the kitten to eat unharassed. A good option with a kitten in a house of older cats is to either separate the kitten at meal times or make an area that is accessible to the kitten but not to the older cats and place the food there. This can be as easy as using a plastic or cardboard box, turning it upside down and cutting a size-appropriate hole in the box. Place the box where it cannot be tipped over, and put the food inside out of reach of the older cats.

TABLE 23.1. **Nutrient profiles.**

KITTEN FOOD DRY

Caloric Distribution (% ME)

Protein: 31%
Fat: 48%
Carbohydrate: 21%
Calories: 568 kcal/cup

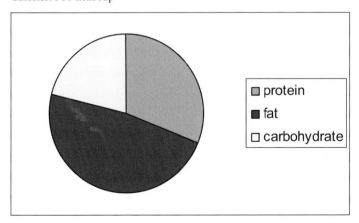

(*Continued*)

TABLE 23.1. (*Continued*)

CAT ADULT MAINTENANCE DRY

Caloric Distribution (% ME)

Protein: 30%
Fat: 46%
Carbohydrate: 24%
Calories: 536 kcal/cup

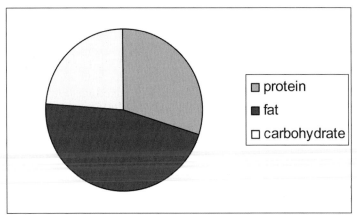

From Eukanuba. 2003. *Veterinary diets product reference guide* (p. 77). Dayton, OH: Iams Co.

Body condition scores should continue to be done, and food intake adjusted to maintain at 3/5 or 4/9 to 5/9 BCS throughout kittenhood and into adulthood. Obesity is much easier to prevent than to treat.

References

Case, L.P., Carey, D.P., Hirakawa, D.A., & Daristotle, L. 2000. Growth. In *Canine and feline nutrition: A resource for companion animal professionals* (2nd. ed., p. 254). St. Louis, MO: Mosby.

Kirk, C.L., Debraekeleer, J., & Armstrong, P.J. 2000. Normal cats. In M.S. Hand, C.D. Thatcher, R.L. Remillard, & P. Roudebush (eds.), *Small animal clinical nutrition* (4th. ed., pp. 247–250). Marceline, MO: Walsworth Publishing for Mark Morris Institute.

LeGrand-Defretin, V., & Munday, H.S. 1995. Feeding dogs and cats for life. In I.H. Burger (ed.), *The Waltham book of companion animal nutrition* (pp. 64–65). Oxford: Butterworth-Heinemann.

24

Adult Maintenance in Dogs

Dogs that have reached mature adult size and are not pregnant, lactating, or working strenuously are defined as being in a state of maintenance (Case et al., 2000). Depending on breed, these are usually dogs between 1 and 7 years of age. Some breeds mature more slowly and do not reach their full mature size until 18 to 24 months of age, while others are full grown by 10 months of age (Case et al., 2000; Gross et al., 2000).

Most companion dogs live indoors in temperate environments. They are usually not pregnant or lactating, not involved in regular work or excessive exercise, and not subject to extremes of temperature (Wills, 1996). For an animal in maintenance, the diet must have the following characteristics (Wills, 1996):

- Provide the correct amount, balance, and availability of nutrients to sustain physical and mental health and activity
- Promote peak condition and therefore reduce its susceptibility to disease
- Be sufficiently nutrient dense to allow the animal to meet its nutrient requirements by eating an amount within the limits set by appetite
- Be sufficiently palatable to ensure an adequate intake

Requirements

The ultimate goals of any maintenance diet are to minimize risk factors for disease and to achieve optimal health. Healthy adult dogs have relatively small nutrient requirements compared with those in the reproductive stages of life. They may be maintained for years on a wide range of diets with few apparent consequences (Buffington et al., 2004). The probability of a diet-related problem should be lower for dogs fed properly formulated commercial diets due to the testing required. Dogs that are fed homemade diets or diets that have not undergone Association of American Feed Control Officials (AAFCO) certification would have significantly higher risks for diet-related problems. Just because an adverse consequence has not been seen in a single animal does not mean that a diet provides superior nutrition (Buffington et al., 2004).

The guidelines printed on pet food labels provide an estimate of the amount of food to feed an average adult dog that is living indoors and provided with moderate amounts of exercise (Case et al., 2000). An estimate of the amount to feed can also be calculated using the dog's ideal body weight, with adjustments in intake being made based on changes in BCS. An animal housed outside of these conditions may require more of less food than recommended. Label guidelines are also based on the food being the only source of nutrition for the dog; this means that no treats, snacks, or table food is being fed. The addition of these foods can significantly change the amount of food that the dog actually requires. Current recommendations are that additional sources of nutrition not compose more than 10% of the entire caloric intake (Gross et al., 2000).

A wide variety of foods is not necessary for most dogs; picky eaters are made by the owner, not by the breeder. Most dogs are best managed on a diet of balanced dog food with a constant supply of fresh, clean water (Case et al., 2000). Frequent changes in the diet can result in gastrointestinal tract upset with resulting diarrhea or vomiting. Sometimes these changes can be seen when feeding a lower-quality commercial brand of food that uses a variable feed formula as opposed to a fixed feed formula. With a variable feed formula, the contents can vary from batch to batch based on market conditions or product availability. As long as the product conforms to the minimums and maximums listed on the guaranteed analysis, the manufacturers can do this. With a fixed feed formula, the ingredients do not change but remain constant from batch to batch. Unfortunately, this information is not listed on the label and can only be obtained by contacting the manufacturer.

Owners should be encouraged to weigh their dog every month or so, with adjustments in intake based on any changes seen. Dogs who are nutritionally well managed are alert, have ideal BCS (3/5 or 4/9 to 5/9) with a stable, normal body weight and a healthy coat. Stools should be firm, well formed, and medium to dark brown in color (Gross et al., 2000).

Stress

Stress can affect the caloric intake of a dog in a number of ways. It is not uncommon for working or boarding dogs to refuse to eat for no apparent reason. Conversely, a dog's appetite may improve with the addition of another dog to the household. If one dog is more dominant and allowed to control access to the food dish, weight loss may be seen in one dog, with weight gain seen in the other (Gross et al., 2000).

Environmental stress can also change energy requirements. In a hot environment, increased water intake can be seen to help with cooling. In colder environments, dogs kept outdoors, even within shelters, need increased energy intake to maintain their body temperatures (Gross et al., 2000). If a change is seen in appetite or BCS, look at possible stressors within the dog's environment.

Obesity

Studies indicate that about 25% of dogs within the United States seen by veterinarians were fat or grossly obese (BCS 4/5 to 5/5 or 7/9 to 9/9) (Burkholder & Toll, 2000). By definition, obesity is the accumulation of an excessive amount of body fat (Burkholder & Toll, 2000). Excess body weight is by far the most prominent form of malnutrition seen in companion animals.

Risk factors associated with obesity include the following (Gross et al., 2000):

• Middle age
• Neuter status
• Low activity
• High-fat, high-calorie foods

Obesity occurs twice as often in neutered dogs than in intact dogs. Neutering does not appear to have a marked impact on resting energy expenditure of female dogs; however, it can significantly increase food intake (Gross et al., 2000). This may be due to a reduction of the appetite-suppressing hormone estrogen (Gross et al., 2000). A decrease in physical activity is also assumed to occur in many dogs after neutering and may play a more important role in male dogs due to decreased roaming (Gross et al., 2000).

It is much easier to prevent an animal from becoming obese than it is to treat obesity once it has occurred. Following BCS in puppyhood to get an adult in the normal-to-lean range is the best way to prevent obesity later in life. True obesity is the direct result of consumption of too much energy.

References

Buffington, T., Holloway, C.A., & Abood, S.K. 2004. Normal dogs. In *Manual of veterinary dietetics* (pp. 15–18). St. Louis, MO: Elsevier.

Burkholder, W.J., & Toll, P.W. 2000. Obesity. In M.S. Hand, C.D. Thatcher, R.L. Remillard, & P. Roudebush (eds.), *Small animal clinical nutrition* (4th. ed., pp. 401–409). Marceline, MO: Walsworth Publishing for Mark Morris Institute.

Case, L.P., Carey, D.P., Hirakawa, D.A., & Daristotle, L. 2000. Adult maintenance. In *Canine and feline nutrition: A resource for companion animal professionals* (2nd. ed., pp. 255–256). St. Louis, MO: Mosby.

Gross, K.L., Wedekind, K.L., Cowell, C.S., Schoenherr,, W.D., Jewell, D.E., Zicker, S.C., Debraekeleer, J., & Frey, R.A. 2000. Normal dogs. In M.S. Hand, C.D. Thatcher, R.L. Remillard, & P. Roudebush (eds.), *Small animal clinical nutrition* (4th. ed., pp. 219–229). Marceline, MO: Walsworth Publishing for Mark Morris Institute.

Wills, J.M. 1996. Adult maintenance. In N.C. Kelly & J.M. Wills (eds.), *Manual of companion animal nutrition and feeding* (pp. 44–46). Ames, IA: Iowa State Press.

25

Adult Maintenance in Cats

Cats that have reached mature adult size and are not pregnant, lactating, or working strenuously are defined as being in a state of maintenance (Case et al., 2000). Cats generally reach adult size between 10 and 12 months of age and reach their full mature weight by 18 months. Adult maintenance is usually the time from 12 months to 8 years (Gross et al., 2000).

Most companion cats live indoors in temperate environments. They are usually not pregnant or lactating, not involved in regular work or excessive exercise, and not subject to extremes of temperature (Wills, 1996). For an animal in maintenance, the diet must have the following characteristics (Wills, 1996):

- Provide the correct amount, balance, and availability of nutrients to sustain physical and mental health and activity
- Promote peak condition and therefore reduce its susceptibility to disease
- Be sufficiently nutrient dense to allow the animal to meet its nutrient requirements by eating an amount within the limits set by appetite
- Be sufficiently palatable to ensure an adequate intake

Requirements

The ultimate goals of any maintenance diet are to minimize risk factors for disease and achieve optimal health and longevity of life. Healthy adult cats have relatively small nutrient requirements compared with those in the reproductive stages of life. They may be maintained for years on a wide range of diets with little apparent consequences (Buffington et al., 2004). The probability of a diet-related problem should be lower for cats fed properly formulated commercial diets due to the testing required. Cats that are fed homemade diets or those that haven't undergone AAFCO certification would pose significantly higher risks for diet-related problems. Just because an adverse consequence has not been seen in a single animal does not mean that a diet provides superior nutrition (Buffington et al., 2004).

The guidelines printed on pet food labels provide an estimate of the amount of food to feed an average adult cat that is living indoors and provided with moderate amounts of exercise (Case et al., 2000). An estimate of the amount to feed can also be calculated using the cat's ideal body weight, with adjustments in intake being made based on changes in BCS. An animal housed outside of these conditions may require more or less food than recommended. Label guidelines are also based on the food being the only source of nutrition for the cat; this means that no treats, snacks, or table food are being fed. The addition of these foods can significantly change the amount of food that the cat actually requires. Current recommendations are that additional sources of nutrition not compose more than 10% of the entire caloric intake (Gross et al., 2000).

A wide variety of foods are not necessary for most cats; picky eaters are not born but are made by the owner. Most cats are best managed on a diet of balanced cat food with a constant supply of fresh, clean water (Case et al., 2000). Frequent changes in the diet can result in gastrointestinal tract upset with resulting diarrhea or vomiting. Sometimes these changes can be seen when feeding a lower-quality commercial brand of food that uses a variable feed formula as opposed to a fixed feed formula. With a variable feed formula, the contents can vary from batch to batch based on market conditions or product availability. As long as the product conforms to the minimums and maximums listed on the guaranteed analysis, the manufacturers can do this. With a fixed feed formula, the ingredients do not change but remain constant from batch to batch. Unfortunately, this information is not listed on the label and can only be obtained by contacting the manufacturer.

Neutering reduces the daily energy requirements by 24% to 33% compared with intact animals (Gross et al., 2000). This decrease does not appear to be affected by age of neutering. The reduction in energy requirements are most likely due to a reduction in basal metabolic rate, because obvious changes in behavior and activity are usually not seen after neutering, especially in young cats (Gross et al., 2000).

By nature, cats do not usually participate in heavy work or endurance-like activities; thus, the variation in energy requirements between active and sedentary cats is small compared with dogs (Gross et al., 2000). Even considering this, a twofold increase can be seen between sedentary and active cats' energy requirements. Food intake should be adjusted according to activity level to maintain a BCS of 3/5 or 4/9 to 5/9.

Sedentary, inactive, caged, or older cats often have energy requirements very near or even below the average resting energy requirement. Cats with unlimited activity may have energy needs 10% to 15% above normal (Gross et al., 2000). Very active or "high-strung" cats may have markedly higher energy expenditures than normal cats, as much as 30% higher than average (Gross et al., 2000).

Although different breeds of cats may have varying nutritional requirements, this variation is less pronounced than that seen with dog breeds (Gross et al., 2000). Some of the more active breeds, such as Abyssinians and Siamese, may have higher energy requirements, whereas others, such as Persians or Rag Dolls, tend to be very tranquil and expend little energy above maintenance (Gross et al., 2000). Disposition tends to affect energy requirements more than does breed.

Cats that are provided proper nutrition are healthy and alert, have ideal body condition and stable weight, and have a clean, glossy hair coat. The owners should ideally evaluate BCS every 2 weeks, monitor daily food and water intake, and observe the cat's interest in food and its appetite. Stools should be evaluated regularly for changes in frequency or character, with normal stools being firm, well formed, and medium to dark brown in color (Gross et al., 2000).

Obesity

By definition, obesity is the accumulation of an excessive amount of body fat (Burkholder & Toll, 2000). Excess body weight is by far the most prominent form of malnutrition seen in companion animals.

Studies indicate that about 25% of cats within the United States seen by veterinarians were fat or grossly obese (BCS 4/5 to 5/5, 7/9 to 9/9)

(Burkholder & Toll, 2000). The highest prevalence being seen in the middle-aged cats (7 to 8 years old) with about 50% of this group being overweight or obese (BCS 4 to 5/5, 7 to 9/9).

Risk factors associated with obesity include:

- Middle age
- Neuter status
- Low activity
- High-fat, high-calorie foods (Gross et al., 2000)

Neutered cats have a resting energy requirement of 20% to 25% less than that of intact cats of a similar age. In practical terms, this means that a neutered cat would require only 75% to 80% of the food required by an intact cat to maintain optimal body condition (Gross et al., 2000).

It is much easier to prevent an obese animal than it is to treat obesity once it has occurred. Following BCS in kittenhood to get an adult in the normal-to-lean range is the best way to prevent obesity later in life. True obesity is the direct result of the consumption of too much energy.

References

Buffington, T., Holloway, C.A., & Abood, S.K. 2004. Nornal dogs. In *Manual of veterinary dietetics* (pp. 30–31). St. Louis, MO: Elsevier.

Burkholder, W.J., & Toll, P.W. 2000. Obesity. In M.S. Hand, C.D. Thatcher, R.L. Remillard, & P. Roudebush (eds.), *Small animal clinical nutrition* (4th. ed., pp. 401–409). Marceline, MO: Walsworth Publishing for Mark Morris Institute.

Case, L.P., Carey, D.P., Hirakawa, D.A., & Daristotle, L. 2000. Adult maintenance. In *Canine and feline nutrition: A resource for companion animal professionals* (2nd. ed., pp. 255–256). St. Louis, MO: Mosby.

Gross, K.L., Wedekind, K.L., Cowell, C.S., Schoenherr,, W.D., Jewell, D.E., Zicker, S.C., Debraekeleer, J., & Frey, R.A. 2000. Normal cats. In M.S. Hand, C.D. Thatcher, R.L. Remillard, & P. Roudebush (eds.), *Small animal clinical nutrition* (4th. ed., pp. 306–314). Marceline, MO: Walsworth Publishing for Mark Morris Institute.

Wills, J.M. 1996. Adult maintenance. In N.C. Kelly & J.M. Wills (eds.), *Manual of companion animal nutrition and feeding* (pp. 44–46). Ames, IA: Iowa State Press.

26

Feeding the Healthy Geriatric Dog and Cat

Continued improvements in control of infection and nutrition in recent years has resulted in a gradual increase in the average life span of the companion cat and dog. The maximum life span of any given species has remained relatively fixed; the average life span within a given population can be affected by genetics, health care, and nutrition (Case et al., 2000). It is estimated that more than 40% of dogs and 30% of cats in the United States are at least 6 years old, and approximately 30% of these animals are older than 11 years (Case et al., 2000).

The average life span of the dog is about 13 years, with a maximal life span of 27 years. Small breeds of dogs tend to live longer than do large and giant breeds (Case et al., 2000).

Cats appear to age more slowly than do dogs and do not show breed differences in aging or longevity (Case et al., 2000). The average life span of the domestic cat is 14 years, with a maximal life span as high as 25 to 35 years. Healthy cats are considered to be geriatric when they are between 10 and 12 years old (Case et al., 2000).

There are breed and size differences at which dogs are considered to be geriatric. The age at which cats are considered geriatric is greater than that for dogs in all categories (Anderson, 1996).

TABLE 26.1. Geriatric onset for cats and dogs.

Category	Body weight in pounds	Age of onset
Small dogs	Under 20 #	11.5 years
Medium dogs	20–50 #	10 years
Large dogs	50–90 #	8.8 years
Giant dogs	Greater than 90 #	7.5 years
Cats		12 years

Feeding Requirements

Although old age is not a disease, there are biologic effects of aging on the body. These include a gradual decline in the functional capacity of organs that begins shortly after the animal has reached maturity (Case et al., 2000). These changes occur in tissue structure and composition, rate of metabolism, cardiovascular and pulmonary function, renal and gastrointestinal tract excretion, special senses, skin, and reproductive system, and virtually all functional and structural systems of the body (Anderson, 1996).

Different systems age at different rates, and the degree of compromise that must occur before the onset of clinical signs also depends on many factors (Case et al., 2000). It is also not unusual for more than one chronic disease to be present in a single geriatric dog or cat (Case et al., 2000). Because of this variability, each older animal should be assessed as an individual, using functional changes in body systems rather than chronological age to assess old age changes (Case et al., 2000).

In dogs and cats, the three leading causes of nonaccidental death are cancer, kidney disease, and heart disease (Gross et al., 2000a).

The objectives for nutritional management of old dogs and cats are as follows (Anderson, 1996; Gross et al., 2000a; Gross et al., 2000b):

- Enhancing the quality of life
- Delaying the onset of aging
- Extending life expectancy
- Slowing or preventing progression of disease
- Eliminating or relieving clinical signs of disease
- Maintaining optimal body condition

Metabolism

Dogs' and cats' metabolism naturally slows as they age, causing a reduction in their resting energy requirement (RER). This decline is due primarily to the loss of lean body mass, even without subsequent loss of body weight (Case et al., 2000). There also tends to be a decrease in activity level as animals age, decreasing their energy output and also decreasing their muscular activity (Anderson, 1996).

The minimum nutrient requirements for older animals are probably similar to those of young to middle-aged animals (Kealy et al., 2002). Because of this, nutritional recommendations for these animals are based on risk factor management, using information obtained on other species, and good sense (Kealy et al., 2002). To date, the only nutritional modification known to slow aging and increase life span is reduction in caloric intake over the life of the animal (Gross et al., 2000b; Kealy et al., 2002). Reducing caloric intake by 20% to 30% of normal while meeting essential nutrient needs reduces the aging process, cancer incidence, occurrence of renal disease, and immune-mediated disease (Gross et al., 2000b; Kealy et al., 2002). This means that animals should be maintained with a BCS of 3/5 or 4/9, significantly lower than what we normally see in our companion animals.

Digestion

There is little to no evidence that healthy older animals are less able to digest their food than younger animals (Anderson, 1996). Digestion and digestibility are therefore not important factors in considering the dietary requirements in most normal dogs and cats (Anderson, 1996). There is no evidence that "geriatric diets" are necessary if the animal is healthy and eating a sufficient amount of a good-quality diet to maintain body weight and body mass (Buffington et al., 2004).

Many geriatric diets are reduced in fat and caloric density to help prevent weight gain as activity level reduces with age. While this may be of benefit to many animals, there are some that have a difficult time maintaining their weight due either to decreased caloric intake or to decreased appetite secondary to various disease processes. It would be prudent to switch these animals to a higher-calorie diet—be it a kitten or puppy diet or, in the case of dogs, a performance diet—to enable them to meet their caloric requirements.

Protein

Due to reduced protein reserves in older animals, avoidance of negative nitrogen balance is important (Anderson, 1996). Dietary protein should not be reduced in apparently healthy older dogs and cats. Adequate protein and energy intake are needed to sustain lean body mass, protein synthesis, and immune function (Gross et al., 2000b). An additional benefit to maintaining moderate protein concentration in foods for older animals is an increase in palatability, which may help maintain an adequate caloric intake (Gross et al., 2000b).

In animals with chronic renal failure, a reduction in dietary protein may be needed to help decrease the serum urea nitrogen (SUN). The kidneys are responsible for excretion of the end-products of protein catabolism; with impaired function, these end-products can accumulate in the bloodstream and cause problems for the animal through the development of uremia (Anderson, 1996; Gross et al., 2000b). Feeding of a protein source with high biologic value will help to decrease the accumulation of these byproducts. The higher the biologic value, the greater is the efficiency of the protein in replenishing or maintaining tissue protein and the less, in proportion to intake, is excreted in the urine as urea (Anderson, 1996). A reduction in protein intake without evidence of chronic renal failure has not been shown to prevent the occurrence of renal failure and may actually cause more problems, such as decreased body mass and decreased body weight due to decreased energy intake and increased protein catabolism of body tissues to meet the animal's protein requirements (Case et al., 2000).

Healthy older animals should receive sufficient protein to adequately meet their protein needs and avoid protein-calorie malnutrition (Gross et al., 2000b). With decreased energy intake, if these older animals are fed a diet that meets the minimum protein requirements for adult animals, they may actually be in a protein deficient (protein-calorie malnutrition) (Case et al., 2000). Therefore, older animals should be fed diets with a percentage of calories from protein slightly higher than the minimum recommended for adult maintenance (Case et al., 2000).

Fat

Fats provide energy, essential fatty acids (EFAs), and a carrier for fat-soluble vitamins and improve the palatability of foods (Anderson, 1996). Because of their high energy density (8.5 kcal/g), the most effective way to affect caloric intake is to modify the fat content of a diet. Although weight loss can be seen in some older animals, obesity by far is the most common problem. It has been theorized that the increase in the percentage of body fat that occurs with aging is partially due to an increased inability of the body to metabolize lipids (Case et al., 2000). There is also evidence that aging is associated with a gradual decline in the ability to desaturate the EFAs (Case et al., 2000).

Certain diseases associated with obesity are also commonly seen in older animals, primarily diabetes mellitus, hypertension, and heart disease, as well as pancreatitis and arthritis (Anderson, 1996; Gross et al., 2000b). The risk of death also increases significantly in older obese animals (Anderson, 1996; Gross et al., 2000b).

Moderate to low levels of fat in the diet are indicated to reduce the risk of obesity or treat obesity that already exists (Gross et al., 2000b). These very same animals may also have impaired fat digestion and fat metabolism. Fats included in foods for older animals should be highly digestible and contain high levels of EFAs. Foods with lower fat levels are recommended for those animals that are obese or obese prone, while foods with higher fat levels should be fed to thin animals (BCS less than 3/5 or 4/9).

Fiber

Dietary fiber promotes gastrointestinal health by aiding normal motility and providing fuel for colonocytes through the production of the fatty acid butyrate. Not all dietary fibers act the same way in the intestines—some are highly digestible and can cause diarrhea (e.g., lactulose), some allow the colonic bacteria to make butyrate (e.g., beet pulp), and some are nondigestible and act as bulking agents (e.g., cellulose) (Anderson, 1996; Gross et al., 2000b).

Many older animals have problems with constipation; this can be treated in one of two ways—by increasing the bulk of the stool to increase frequency of defecation or by feeding a low-fiber food to increase digestibility and decrease stool volume and therefore colonic distention (Case et al., 2000; Gross et al., 2000b). In refractory cases, lactulose may be added to the diet to increase the amount of water in the colon, keeping the stool moister and making it easier to defecate. As it is difficult to tell which method will work best for any individual animal, all three methods may need to be tried.

Conclusion

Many older animals become very particular about their eating habits. There may be a decreased willingness to eat new foods, and it may be necessary for the owners to provide especially strong smelling or highly palatable foods (Case et al., 2000). The animals may also develop very fixed food preferences; if possible, owners should

TABLE 26.2. **Practical feeding tips for geriatric dogs and cats.**

- Provide regular geriatric health exams at least twice yearly
- Avoid sudden changes in daily routine or diet
- Feed a diet that contains high-quality protein specifically formulated for geriatric animals
- Use measured feedings to help prevent obesity and maintain ideal body weight
- Provide a moderate amount of regular exercise
- Maintain proper dental health with home care and regular dental cleanings
- If needed, provide a therapeutic diet to help manage or treat a disease

accommodate these if the food provides adequate nutrition to the animal (Case et al., 2000).

If a chronic disease is present that requires specific nutrient alterations such as diabetes, renal disease, arthritis, or obesity, the animal should be fed a diet that is appropriate for the management of that disorder. If multiple diseases are present, feed for the most life-threatening disease (Case et al., 2000).

Proper care of teeth and gums is especially important as animals age; if their mouths hurt or are a source of bacteria, this can negatively affect their overall health. If owners are unable or unwilling to provide at-home dental care, yearly to biyearly oral health care should be done through the veterinarian (Case et al., 2000).

Exercise is also important in the older animal to help maintain muscle tone, enhance circulation, improve gastrointestinal motility, and prevent excess weight gain. The level and intensity of the exercise should be adjusted to an individual animal's physical and medical condition (Case et al., 2000).

References

Anderson, R.S. 1996. Feeding older pets. In N.C. Kelly & J.M. Wills (eds.), *Manual of companion animal nutrition and feeding* (pp. 93–98). Ames, IA: Iowa State Press.

Buffington, T., Holloway, C.A., & Abood, S.K. 2004. Normal dogs. In *Manual of veterinary dietetics* (pp. 21–23). St. Louis, MO: Elsevier.

Case, L.P., Carey, D.P., Hirakawa, D.A., & Daristotle, L. 2000. Geriatrics. In *Canine and feline nutrition: A resource for companion animal professionals* (2nd. ed., pp. 275–286). St. Louis, MO: Mosby.

Gross, K.L., Wedekind, K.L., Cowell, C.S., Schoenherr,, W.D., Jewell, D.E., Zicker, S.C., Debraekeleer, J., & Frey, R.A. 2000a. Normal dogs. In M.S. Hand, C.D. Thatcher, R.L. Remillard, & P. Roudebush (eds.), *Small animal clinical nutrition* (4th. ed., pp. 229–232). Marceline, MO: Walsworth Publishing for Mark Morris Institute.

Gross, K.L., Debraekeleer, J., & Zicker, S.C. 2000b. Normal cats. In M.S. Hand, C.D. Thatcher, R.L. Remillard, & P. Roudebush (eds.), *Small animal clinical nutrition* (4th. ed., pp. 314–320). Marceline, MO: Walsworth Publishing for Mark Morris Institute.

Kealy, R.D., Lawler, D.F., Ballam, J.M., Mantz, S.L., Biery, D.N., Greeley, E.H., Lust, G., Segre, M., Smith, G.K., & Stowe, H.D. 2002. Effects of diet restriction on life span and age-related changes in dogs. *Journal of the American Veterinary Medical Association, 220,* 1315–1320.

27

Performance and Dogs

People have spent much time and energy over the years molding dogs into various shapes to suit our needs; the *Illustrated Encyclopedia of Dog Breeds* lists 91 hound breeds, 43 working breeds, 44 herding breeds, 49 gun dogs, and 31 terrier breeds (Toll & Reynolds, 2000). Due to our changing lifestyle, many of these breeds are no longer needed for what they were bred. These breeds still contain the genetic makeup for their original activities; this means that many of our companions have much more energy than is needed for a couch potato.

Working dogs are still found in many areas. The federal, local, and state governments employ dogs in areas of national defense, customs service, and border patrol. Dogs are trained for service animals for the deaf and blind, as well as the physically disabled. They are also still used for hunting, racing, endurance sled pulling, and other athletic competitions. Canine agility competitions, Frisbee competitions, and herding competitions are found in many parts of our country. These provide a wonderful opportunity for human and dog to work together again as they were originally trained without having to maintain a herd of sheep!

Just like people who are athletes, training and nutrition can play a major role in the canine athletes' success. But nutrition cannot overcome deficits in genetics and training. Matching nutrition to exercise type allows a canine athlete to perform to its genetic potential and level of training (Toll & Reynolds, 2000). In general, all working dogs have increased energy requirements over those of an adult dog during time of normal activity (Case et al., 2000). The type of work being done and the intensity of work may require modifications in the nutrient composition of the food and the feeding schedule (Case et al., 2000).

The work performed by most intermediate athletes (hunting dogs, field trials, Frisbee trials, agility, service work, police work, search and rescue, livestock management, and exercise with people) resembles that done by endurance athletes (sled pulling) but is of shorter duration. The muscle fiber type profile of intermediate athletes should resemble that of an endurance athlete over that of a sprint athlete (sight hounds) (Case et al., 2000). In general, endurance athletes have an increased number of well-developed slow-twitch fiber muscles; athletes involved in high-speed sprinting have increased numbers of fast-twitch muscles (Case et al., 2000). Slow-twitch muscles have a higher capacity for aerobic metabolism, meaning that they primarily use fat in the form of free fatty acids for energy. Fast-twitch muscles can use both aerobic and anaerobic pathways in that they can use both carbohydrates in the form of glycogen and glucose for immediate energy and fat for longer-term energy use (Case et al., 2000; Toll & Reynolds, 2000).

Exercise requires transfer of chemical energy into physical work. ATP (adenosine triphosphate) is the sole source of energy for muscle contraction (Toll & Reynolds, 2000). ATP is formed from metabolic fuels stored in muscle (endogenous) and from other body stores (exogenous). The energy is converted to ATP via either aerobic pathways that use oxygen or anaerobic pathways that can work without oxygen (Toll & Reynolds, 2000). The proportion of each pathway used is determined by duration and intensity of exercise, conditioning, and nutritional status of the animal (Toll & Reynolds, 2000).

Training and conditioning result in adaptive physiological changes that facilitate efficient delivery of oxygen and other nutrients to the working muscle. Some of these changes include increased blood volume, increased red blood cell mass, increased capillary density, increased mitochondrial volume, increased activity, and total mass of metabolic enzymes (Case et al., 2000).

Fats

The two primary fuels used by the body for working muscles are muscle glycogen and free fatty acids. An intermediate athlete would receive about 70% to 90% of their energy from fat metabolism and only a small amount from carbohydrate metabolism (Case et al., 2000). Dogs rely more heavily on free fatty acids for energy generation at all exercise levels than do people (Toll & Reynolds, 2000). Feeding a higher-fat diet to endurance and intermediate trained athletes prepares the muscles to efficiently mobilize and use free fatty acids for energy. It also exerts a glycogen-sparing effect that can help prolong glycogen use during work (Case et al., 2000). By increasing dietary fat concentration, you can increase the energy intake and encourage stressed dogs to increase food intake due to the increased palatability of fat in the diet (Toll & Reynolds, 2000). Increased dietary fat levels may also enhance free fatty acid availability (Toll & Reynolds, 2000).

Carbohydrate

Provided sufficient gluconeogenic precursors are available in the diet, no dietary requirements for carbohydrates exist except during gestation and neonatal development (Toll & Reynolds, 2000). Gluconeogenesis (formation of glucose from noncarbohydrate sources) is performed by the liver and kidneys using glycerol, lactate, and glucogenic amino acids (Toll & Reynolds, 2000). Adipose tissue supplies glycerol for glucose production, breaking down triglycerides and fatty acids for oxidation to supply energy, whereas muscle catabolism releases glucogenic amino acids, lactic acid, and pyruvate for glucose production by the liver (Toll & Reynolds, 2000).

Carbohydrates fed to athletes should be highly digestible to decrease fecal bulk in the colon. Excessive amounts of undigested carbohydrates reaching the colon can increase water loss through the stool, increase colonic gas production, and increase overall fecal bulk and therefore add unneeded weight (Toll & Reynolds, 2000).

Protein

Endurance training results in increased protein needs through increased protein synthesis (anabolism [the building up of muscle]) and protein degradation (catabolism [the breaking down of muscle]) (Case et al., 2000; Toll & Reynolds, 2000). Catabolism is only a small portion of the overall protein needs; the primary use is anabolism (Case et al., 2000). Increased tissue mass associated with training must be supplied by increased protein in the diet (Case et al., 2000). Amino acids are used in the formation of new muscle and repair damage to muscle and connective tissue during intensive conditioning; exercise increases the amino acid catabolism (Toll & Reynolds, 2000).

Amino acids provide about 5% to 15% of the energy used during exercise; most of this energy comes from the branched-chain amino acids (leucine, isoleucine, and valine). All of these are essential amino acids and cannot be synthesized from other amino acids; they must be included in the diet. The "biologic value" of a protein is an indicator of the amount of essential amino acids found in that product. Muscle- and organ meat–based proteins have the highest level of essential amino acids and are also the most digestible and most bioavailable.

Excessive protein intake may predispose an athlete to increased amino acid catabolism. Amino acids are not stored as proteins in the body but are deaminated (broken down) to ketoacids. These ketoacids are either oxidized for energy or converted to fatty acids and/or glucose and stored as adipose tissue (fat) or glycogen (Toll & Reynolds, 2000). The diet fed should supply adequate calories as fat and carbohydrate so that the protein fed can be used primarily for tissue synthesis and not for energy (Case et al., 2000).

Water

Water is used as a solvent for biological solutes; it acts as a transport medium for nutrients, wastes, and heat; absorbs physical shock; and lubricates various internal and external surfaces (Toll & Reynolds, 2000). Heat is the primary byproduct of muscle contraction, and the respiratory tract, through panting, is responsible for dissipation of this heat (Toll & Reynolds, 2000). Because evaporative heat loss is the primary way in which dogs dissipate heat, ensuring adequate hydration is crucial for the maintenance of normal body temperature (Toll & Reynolds, 2000). Depending on the type of work done and environmental conditions, water losses can increase by 10 to 20 times normal during exercise (Case et al., 2000). Even mild dehydration can lead to decreased performance, decreased strength, and hyperthermia (Case et al., 2000). Water should be offered in small amounts frequently throughout the exercise period. If an insufficient amount is consumed, the dog might benefit by having water added to its food (Toll & Reynolds, 2000).

Supplements

Many breeders, exhibitors, and trainers believe stressed dogs must also receive supplements of certain vitamins and minerals. There is no evidence to suggest that working dogs have increased requirements of these nutrients (Case et al., 2000). If a diet is nutritionally balanced and the dog is consuming enough to meet its energy requirements during work, then additional supplements should not be necessary (Toll & Reynolds, 2000).

Diet Requirements

A diet needs to be highly digestible to limit the total volume of food consumed at each meal. Some maintenance diets may supply enough energy if consumed in large enough quantities, but may become bulk limiting and thereby limit performance in hard working dogs (too much stool production due to low digestibility) (Case et al., 2000).

An ideal diet would provide increased levels of high-quality protein to meet anabolic requirements and enough nonprotein energy nutrients (fats and carbohydrates) to meet energy requirements. By doing this, the diet provides sufficient calories with fat to limit the use of amino acids for energy, leaving them available for muscle repair and replacement (Case et al., 2000).

The food needs to be calorically dense and palatable, highly digestible, and practical, so that the dog can physically consume enough to meet its caloric requirements (Toll & Reynolds, 2000). The price of the food, the form in which it is available, storage conditions required, and number of animals being fed also need to be taken into account. What may be practical for one dog may be impractical for a kennel of 15 dogs (Toll & Reynolds, 2000).

Diet Considerations

Daily energy requirements (DER) can be highly variable and are directly related to the amount of work being done and the condition and training of the dog. Ambient temperature, psychological stress, and geography are all environmental factors that may influence nutritional needs of the canine athlete (Toll & Reynolds, 2000). Of these, ambient temperature can exert the greatest effect; with increased environmental temperature, you get increased work and increased water loss. Lower environmental temperature increases energy expenditure for thermogenesis; this may be as much as a 50% increase over DER (Case et al., 2000; Toll & Reynolds, 2000).

Stress in the form of intense physical exertion, weather extremes, and psychological strain may negatively affect food intake, and an adequate amount of energy may not be available for the work required

(Case et al., 2000; Toll & Reynolds, 2000). Geographical factors such as elevation above sea level and changing elevations throughout a course, as well as working in sand or tall grass, may increase the workload and thereby energy expenditure (Toll & Reynolds, 2000).

Diet Calculations

The amount of energy required depends on the total work done: intensity × duration × frequency. DER is approximately 1.6 × RER (resting energy requirements) for the average canine athlete. Sprinters may require 1.6 to 2 × RER, and endurance or other high-end athletes may require 2 to 5 × RER.

Resting energy requirements can either be figured using 70 × body weight in kilograms (0.75 power), or 70 + (30 × body weight in kilograms). From there you can calculate the DER. Maintenance is typically 1.0 to 1.6 × RER depending on activity.

Feeding Plan

Look at where the dog is housed (inside or outside), medications it may be taking, dietary history, amount fed, type of food fed, timing of meals in relation to exercise and training and the nutrient profile of the diet, and exercise and training history (amount of exercise done, frequency and performance of exercise) (Toll & Reynolds, 2000).

Compare the current diet's key nutritional factors, and determine the amount to be fed and the timing of the meals. Estimate energy expenditure using body condition scoring and exercise level.

Timing of meals is important to allow the most availability of nutrients to the athlete. The ideal plan is one meal at least 4 hours before exercise, one meal within 2 hours after exercise, and, if necessary, due to the duration of exercise, small amounts during exercise. The largest meal should be given after exercise. It is also very important to allow access to plenty of cool, fresh, clean water to prevent dehydration (Toll & Reynolds, 2000).

Reassess your plan based on body condition scoring, weight, hydration, and performance. Adjust as needed to get the results that you want from your canine athlete.

The list in Table 27.1 represents products with the largest market share and for which published information is available. Values are expressed in percentage of metabolizable energy (ME) (Toll & Reynolds, 2000).

TABLE 27.1 **Products with the largest market share and for which published information is available.**

Food	ME Protein	ME Fat	ME Carbohydrate
Diamond Professional Dog Food, dry	28%	45%	27%
Dr. Ballard Great Performance, dry	26%	50%	24%
Eagle Pack Kennel, dry	25%	35%	40%
Eagle Pack Power pack, dry	28%	44%	28%
Hill's Science Diet Canine Active Adult, dry	23%	50%	26%
Hill's Science Diet Canine Active Adult, canned	23%	49%	28%
Iams Eukanuba Premium Performance, dry	27%	48%	28%
Nutro's Natural Choice Plus, dry	27%	41%	32%
Pedigree Chum Advance Formula Activity Plus, dry	29%	44%	27%
Purina Hi Pro, dry	28%	26%	46%
Purina Pro Plan Performance, dry	28%	42%	30%
Royal Canin HE30, dry	29%	38%	33%
Royal Canin ST35, dry	30%	53%	17%
Wafcol Energy Plus, dry	27%	25%	48%

Adapted from Toll, P.W., & Reynolds, A.J. 2000. The canine athlete. In M.S. Hand, C.D. Thatcher, R.L. Remillard, & P. Roudebush (eds.), *Small animal clinical nutrition* (4th. ed., pp. 261–283). Marceline, MO: Walsworth Publishing for Mark Morris Institute.

To express nutrients as a percentage of ME, see Table 27.2.

Comparing products using ME gives a better idea of caloric distribution and allows you to accurately compare canned and dry diets. This does not take into account digestibility. It is also important when

TABLE 27.2. **Total calories in 100 g of food.**

Protein = 3.5 kcal/gram × grams in food
Fat = 8.5 kcal/gram × grams in food
Carbohydrate = 3.5 kcal/gram × grams in food
Total calories/100 g = protein calorie + fat calorie + carbohydrate calorie

Percentage of ME contributed by each nutrient (caloric distribution)
Protein = (protein calories/100 g divided by total calories/100 g) × 100 = % ME
Fat = (fat calories/100 g divided by total calories/100 g) × 100 = % ME
Carbohydrate = (carbohydrate calories/100 g divided by total calories)
× 100 = % ME

TABLE 27.3. **Recommended caloric distribution for canine athletes.**

Calories from protein: 30–35% ME
Calories from fat: 50–65% ME
Calories from carbohydrate: 10–15% ME

From Case, L.P., Carey, D.P., Hirakawa, D.A., & Daristotle, L. 2000a. Performance and stress. In *Canine and feline nutrition: A resource for companion animal professionals* (2nd. ed., pp. 259–273). St. Louis, MO: Mosby.

comparing foods to see if feeding trials have been done on the product and to look at digestibility, if given. If you chose a food that has not had feeding trials done by the manufacturer, then you are doing the feeding trials for them.

References

Case, L.P., Carey, D.P., Hirakawa, D.A., & Daristotle, L. 2000. Performance and stress. In *Canine and feline nutrition: A resource for companion animal professionals* (2nd. ed., pp. 259–273). St. Louis, MO: Mosby.
Toll, P.W., & Reynolds, A.J. 2000. The canine athlete. In M.S. Hand, C.D. Thatcher, R.L. Remillard, & P. Roudebush (eds.), *Small animal clinical nutrition* (4th. ed., pp. 261–283). Marceline, MO: Walsworth Publishing for Mark Morris Institute.

28

Nutritional Requirements of Cats

In their natural environment, cats are an obligate carnivore, meaning that their nutritional needs are met by eating a diet that consists of animal-based proteins (e.g., mice, birds). How have our efforts to domesticate cats been affected by this dietary requirement?

Strictly speaking, cats and dogs are members of the order Carnivora and are therefore classified as carnivores. From a dietary perspective, dogs are omnivores and cats and other members of the suborder Felidae are strict carnivores. Domesticated cats *(Felis catus)* have evolved unique anatomic, physiologic, metabolic, and behavioral adaptations consistent with eating a strictly carnivorous diet (Case et al., 2000; Kirk et al., 2000).

Feeding Behaviors

The evolutionary history of the cat indicates that it has eaten a purely carnivorous diet throughout its entire development (Kirk et al., 2000). Feeding behaviors that have evolved to fit this lifestyle include searching, hunting, and catching of prey as well as postprandial behaviors such as grooming and sleeping (Voith, 1994). Feral or outdoor cats feeding primarily on mice, voles, and insects tend to live solitary lives when food is scarce and spread over a large area, but when food is plentiful and concentrated as with households, dumps, and farms, cats can be found living in large groups (Voith, 1994). Cats typically eat 10 to 20 small meals throughout the day and night. This eating pattern probably reflects the relationship between cats and their prey. Small rodents make up about 40% or more of the feral domestic cat's diets, with small rabbits, insect, frogs, and birds composing the remainder. The average mouse provides about 30 kcal, or an estimated 8% of a feral cat's daily energy requirements. Repeated cycles of hunting throughout the day and night are required to provide sufficient food for the average cat (Case et al., 2000; Kirk et al., 2000). House cats typically continue this pattern by eating 10 to 20 small meal throughout the day and night, with each meal having a caloric content of about 23 kcal, very close to the caloric value of one small mouse (Case et al., 2000; Kirk et al., 2000).

For thousands of years, the primary economic value of cats has been their hunting skills (Voith, 1994). Until recently, there has been little or no selective breeding done to alter their behavior or looks. The predatory drive is so strong in cats that they will stop eating to make a kill. This behavior allows for multiple kills, which optimizes food availability (Kirk et al., 2000). Supplemental feeding may reduce the time spent hunting but otherwise will not alter hunting behavior (Kirk et al., 2000).

Cats are very sensitive to the physical form, odor, and taste of foods. They consume live prey beginning at the head; this head-first consumption is dictated by the direction of hair growth on the prey (Kirk et al., 2000). Food temperature also influences acceptance by cats. They do not readily accept food served at either temperature extreme but prefer food near body temperature (about 38 °C [101.5 °F]), as would be found with freshly killed prey (Kirk et al., 2000; Voith, 1994). House cats accustomed to a specific texture or type of food may refuse foods with different textures. An individual cat's preferences are often influenced by early experiences (good or bad). Many cats will choose a new food over a diet that is currently being fed. The reverse is true in new or stressful situations, such as illness or hospitalization, where cats tend to refuse novel foods. This can be important to know when trying to switch foods or forms of food fed (Kirk et al., 2000).

Anatomic Adaptations

Cats have adapted physiologically to the life of a hunter. Their visual acuity is greater than that of dogs. In addition, their sense of hearing is well developed—their ears are upright, face forward, and they have 20 associated muscles to help them precisely locate sound. Their highly sensitive facial whiskers and widely dispersed tactile hairs are thought to help them hunt in dim light and protect their eyes (Kirk et al., 2000). Sharp and dagger-like, their retractable claws are ideal for capturing and securing prey, yet they are easily retracted to decrease noise when stalking (Kirk et al., 2000).

The scissors-like carnassial teeth are ideal for delivering the cervical bite used to severe the spinal cord and immobilize or kill prey (Kirk et al., 2000).

Their stomachs are smaller than dogs and simpler in structure. Because cats do not consume large meals, the stomach is less important as a storage reservoir (Kirk et al., 2000).

Intestinal length, as determined by the ratio of intestine to body length, is markedly shorter in cats than in omnivores and herbivores. The ratio for cats is 4:1, meaning that the intestinal length is four times longer than the length of the cat; for dogs, this is 6:1, and for pigs, 14:1 (Kirk et al., 2000). Cats do have greater villus height in their intestinal lining, improving their absorptive capacity over that of dogs, so that overall they are only about 10% less efficient in digestion, especially with complex starches or fibers, even with their shorter intestinal length (Kirk et al., 2000).

Physiologic Adaptations

Cats are not able to adapt to varying levels of carbohydrates in their diets due to various changes in the digestive and absorptive functions of intestine. Salivary amylase, the enzyme used to initiate digestion of dietary starches, is absent in cats, and intestinal amylase appears to be exclusively derived from the pancreas. These enzymes were not necessary in a prey-based diet with minimal starch content (Kirk et al., 2000). The level of pancreatic amylase is only 5% that of dogs. The sugar transporter in the intestine is nonadaptive to changes in dietary carbohydrate levels. Disaccharide activity (i.e., the brush border enzymes responsible for sugar digestion) is also nonadaptive and only about 40% that found in dogs (Kirk et al., 2000; Zoran, 2002). These changes evolved because cats had little natural carbohydrate intake and it was not necessary to have systems intact that were of little use to the animal.

Despite these adaptive changes, cats are able to still use carbohydrates in their diets, with a sugar digestibility of about 94% with a few exceptions. Lactose digestion declines sharply in kittens after 7 weeks of age. This is due to a decrease in intestinal lactase activity that is typical in mammals. Most adult cats can consume small amounts of milk without problems, but larger amounts (>1.3 g/kg body weight) can lead to signs of bloating, diarrhea, and gas (Kirk et al., 2000).

High amounts of dietary carbohydrate levels can negatively affect diet digestibility. With high levels of dietary carbohydrates, decreases in protein digestibility are seen due to a combination of factors, including reduced fecal pH caused by incomplete carbohydrate digestion and increased microbial fermentation in the colon with increased production of organic acids (Kirk et al., 2000; Zoran, 1994). Cats have a vestigial cecum and short colon, which limit their ability to use poorly digestible starches and fiber for energy through bacterial fermentation in the large bowel (Kirk et al., 2000).

Metabolic Adaptations

Energy

The liver of most animals has two active enzyme systems for converting glucose to glucose-6-phosphate (the first step to forming glycogen, the storage form of glucose within the cells), hexokinase, and glucokinase (Welborn & Moldawer, 1997). The glucokinase system is used primarily when a large load of glucose is received by the liver as would be seen with a high-carbohydrate meal. Cats have very low liver glucokinase activity and therefore limited ability to metabolize large amounts of simple carbohydrates via this route. Blood glucose levels in carnivores are more consistent with less postprandial fluctuations because glucose is released in small continuous boluses over a longer period of time as a result of gluconeogenic catabolism of proteins (Kirk et al., 2000). If the protein is not included in the diet, body muscle and organ tissue will be used. Cats did not need to handle large carbohydrate loads and therefore only use the hexokinase system for glucose metabolism.

Water

Domestic cats are thought to have descended from the small African wildcat *(Felis silvestris libyca),* a cat naturally found in the deserts of Africa. Because of this ancient relationship, cats today maintain this adaptation to a dryer environment. Cats seem to be less sensitive to the stimulus of thirst and are able to survive on less water than can dogs (Case et al., 2000; Kirk et al., 2000; Zoran, 2002).

With this decreased response to thirst, cats may ignore minor levels of dehydration (up to 4% body weight). They are able to compensate for this reduced water intake by forming highly concentrated urine (Zoran,

2002). Cats adjust their water intake based on the dry matter content of their diet rather than the moisture content. They consume 1.5 to 2 ml of water/g of dry matter. This 2:1 ratio of water to dry matter is similar to that of their typical prey (Kirk et al., 2000; Zoran, 2002). Practically, this means that cats consuming a dry food diet will consume about half the amount of water through their diet and drinking, compared with cats eating a canned food diet (Kirk et al., 2000; Zoran, 2002).

Protein

Protein metabolism in cats is unique; this is apparent because of their unusually high maintenance requirement for protein in the diet compared with dogs or other omnivores. Cats have both a higher basal requirement for protein and an increased requirement for essential amino acids (Voith, 1994). Cats depend on protein not only for structural and synthetic purposes but also for energy. They will continue to use protein in the form of gluconeogenic amino acids for production of energy, even when inadequate protein is consumed in the diet (Kirk et al., 2000). Although these changes impair the cat's ability to conserve protein when dietary sources are limited, on their natural diet, ultimately energy is conserved by eliminating the cost of enzyme synthesis and degradation (Kirk et al., 2000).

In 1986, the National Research Council (NRC) recommended a minimum of 240 g of protein/kg in the diets of growing kitten and 140g of protein/kg in the diets of adult cats. This is equivalent to 26% of metabolizable energy in the diet for kittens and 23% of metabolizable energy for adult maintenance. Keep in mind, these are minimum recommendations, and they assume a highly digestible protein source is provided in the diet.

Taurine

Taurine, which is an essential amino acid for cats, is not incorporated into proteins or degraded by mammalian tissues, but is essential for conjugation of bile salts, vision, cardiac muscle function, and proper function of the nervous, reproductive, and immune systems (Voith, 1994; Wills, 1996; Zoran, 2002). Cats can only conjugate bile acids with taurine to make bile salts. Taurine continues to be lost in the gastrointestinal tract through this conjugation with bile; this coupled with a low rate of synthesis contributes to the obligatory requirement for cats (Kirk et al., 2000; Voith, 1994; Wills, 1996; Zoran, 2002). A carnivorous diet supplies abundant taurine; however, cereals and grains supply only marginal or inadequate levels of taurine for cats (Voith, 1994). Therefore, diets based on these types of protein sources may be lacking or limited in taurine. Taurine is either more available or better retained by cats fed dry food diets.

Because of the widespread uses of taurine within the body, changes from deficiency can be seen in virtually all body systems (Voith, 1994). Three syndromes have been identified related strictly to taurine deficiency: feline central retinal degeneration, reproductive failure and impaired fetal development, and feline dilated cardiomyopathy (Kirk et al., 2000). Clinical signs of taurine deficiency occur only after prolonged periods of depletion (from 5 months to 2 years) (Kirk et al., 2000).

Methionine and Cystine

Methionine is an essential amino acid for cats, which have a higher requirement than do dogs or other omnivores. Cystine is also required for production of hair and felinine, an amino acid found in cat urine. Felinine is found in largest amounts in intact male cats and is thought to be used for territorial marking (Kirk et al., 2000; Zoran, 2002). Cystine can replace up to half of the methionine requirement in cats; methionine tends to be the first limiting amino acid in many food ingredients (Kirk et al., 2000).

Nutritional deficiencies are possible, especially in cats fed homemade, vegetable-based diets or human enteral diets. Clinical signs of methionine deficiency include poor growth and a crusting dermatitis at the mucocutaneous junctions of the mouth and nose (Kirk et al., 2000; Zoran, 2002).

Vitamin Metabolism

The cat is unable to convert beta-carotene to retinol (vitamin A) because of a lack of intestinal enzymes necessary for the conversion, and therefore this species requires a dietary source of preformed vitamin A. Vitamin A is necessary for the maintenance of vision, bone and muscle growth, reproduction, and healthy epithelial tissues. Because vitamin A is a fat-soluble vitamin and is stored in the liver, deficiencies are slow to develop and are only seen in cats with severe liver failure or gastrointestinal disease resulting in fat malabsorption (Zoran, 2002). Cats also are unable to convert sufficient amounts of the fatty acid linoleic acid to meet the requirements for arachidonic acid (Kirk et al., 2000; Wills, 1996; Zoran, 2002).

Cats also lack sufficient enzymes to meet the metabolic requirements for vitamin D photosynthesis in the skin; therefore, they require a dietary source of vitamin D (Kirk et al., 2000). The primary function of vitamin D is calcium and phosphorus homeostasis, with particular emphasis on intestinal absorption, retention, and bone deposition of calcium (Zoran, 2002). As with vitamin A, deficiency is rare and slow to develop (Kirk et al., 2000; Zoran, 2002).

Vitamin A, vitamin D, and arachidonic acid are found in plentiful amounts in animal fats. This fat is important not only for provision of fuel for energy but also for increasing palatability and acceptance of food (Zoran, 2002).

Cats require increased amounts of many dietary water-soluble B vitamins, including thiamin, niacin, pyridoxine (vitamin B6), and, in certain circumstances, cobalamin (vitamin B12). The requirement for niacin and pyridoxine is four times higher than that for dogs (Kirk et al., 2000; Zoran, 2002). Because most water-soluble B vitamins are not stored (except cobalamin, which is stored in the liver), a continually available dietary source is required to prevent deficiencies (Voith, 1994). Deficiencies are rare in cats eating appropriate diets because each of the B vitamins is found in high concentrations in animal tissue (Zoran, 2002).

Conclusion

The cat may be seen as one of our most visible "specialists." As an obligate carnivore, they have evolved to such a point that many of the redundant systems that we have are no longer required. Instead of seeing cats as "inferior," we need to acknowledge that they have surpassed both humans and dogs and have streamlined their lives. We need to appreciate this unique and wonderful creature that continues to enrich our lives and protect our houses and yards.

References

Case, L.P., Carey, D.P., Hirakawa, D.A., & Daristotle, L. 2000. Nutritional idiosyncrasies for cats. In *Canine and feline nutrition: A resource for companion animal professionals* (2nd. ed., pp. 71–73). St. Louis, MO: Mosby.

Kirk, C.L., Debraekeleer, J., & Armstrong, P.J. 2000. Normal cats. In M.S. Hand, C.D. Thatcher, R.L. Remillard, & P. Roudebush (eds.), *Small animal clinical nutrition* (4th. ed., pp. 291–337). Marceline, MO: Walsworth Publishing for Mark Morris Institute.

Voith, V. 1994. Feeding behaviors. In J.M. Wills & K.W. Simpson (eds.), *Waltham book of clinical nutrition of the dog and cat* (pp. 119–127). Tarrytown, NY: Pergamon Press.

Welborn, M.B., & Moldawer, L.L. 1997. Glucose metabolism. In J.L. Rombeau & R.H. Rollandelli (eds.), *Clinical nutrition: Enteral and tube feeding* (pp. 61–80). Philadelphia: W.B. Saunders.

Wills, J.M. 1996. Adult maintenance. In N.C. Kelly & J.M. Wills (eds.), *Manual of companion animal nutrition and feeding* (pp. 44–46). Ames, IA: Iowa State Press.

Zoran, D.L. 2002. The carnivore connection to nutrition in cats. *Journal of the American Veterinary Medical Association, 221,* 1559–1566.

29

Nutrition Myths

With the ready availability of the Internet, clients have an even greater access to information. Where previously they had relied on information from their friends, breeders, and news sources, now they can add the "Net" to their source network. Unfortunately, they do not tend to "filter" out the information, taking everything in their source network as gospel, and do not look at the source or references. Many clients feel uncomfortable talking to their veterinarian about nutrition questions or feel that they know as much as the veterinarian does. This has led many a good-intentioned client to follow poor recommendations. Some of the more common "myths" are presented below, followed by the truth.

Myth: Meat Byproducts Are Inferior in Quality Compared with Whole Meat in a Diet

When listed on an ingredient label, "meat" is defined by the Association of American Feed Control Officials (AAFCO) as any combination of skeletal striated muscle or that muscle found in the tongue, diaphragm, heart, or esophagus with or without the accompanying and overlying fat and the portions of the skin, sinew, nerve, and blood vessels that normally accompany the muscle derived from part of whole carcasses. It also must be suitable for use in animal foods. This excludes feathers, heads, feet, and entrails (Gross et al., 2000a, 2000b, 2000c). "Meat byproducts" are defined as nonrendered, clean parts of the carcass that may contain lungs, spleen, kidneys, brain, liver, blood, bone, heads, feet (of poultry), partially defatted fatty tissue, stomach, and intestines emptied of their contents. It does not include hair, horns, teeth, or hooves (Gross et al., 2000a, 2000b, 2000c). Depending on the supplier and the type of refining process that the manufacturer uses, byproducts can vary greatly in the amount of nondigestible material they contain. The ash content can give you an idea of the quality of the byproducts. High ash content is an indicator of a poorer-quality protein with lesser digestibility. The presence of byproducts does not indicate a poor-quality diet; a higher ash-to-protein ratio would indicate this. Feeding trials evaluating nutrient content and digestibility will help greatly in evaluating the quality of the ingredients. This information is available in most product reference guides, online references, and by contacting the manufacturer. Knowing the reputation of the manufacturer is your best indicator of a good quality diet.

Myth: Feeding Trials Are Not Necessary

Feeding trial protocol as established by the AAFCO for adult maintenance lasts 6 months, requires only eight animals per group, and monitors a limited number of parameters. These parameters are set at the minimum nutrient requirements as defined by the National Research Council (NRC) (Case et al., 2000a, 2000b; Gross et al., 2000a, 2000b, 2000c). These levels tend to be lower than the recommended daily intake (RDI). Requirements are the minimum level of a nutrient that over time is sufficient to maintain the desired physiological functions of the animals in the population. RDI is the level of intake of a nutrient that appears to be adequate to meet known nutritional needs of practically all healthy individuals. The NRC recommendations are to serve as a guide to diet formulations, but they do not account for digestibility or nutrient availability. AAFCO feeding trials provide reasonable assurance of nutrient availability and sufficient palatability to ensure acceptability. They also provide some assurance that the product will support certain functions such as gestation, lactation, and growth (Gross et al., 2000a, 2000b, 2000c). A feeding trial is also the only way to accurately access the quality of the protein in a diet, as this is the only valid way to determine digestibility of a protein, and therefore its quality. Passing a feeding trial does not ensure that the food will be effective in preventing long-term nutrition and health problems or in detecting problems with a low prevalence in the general population. A feeding trial is also not designed to ensure optimal growth or maximize physical activity. If a diet has not gone through a feeding trial by the manufacturer, you will be conducting the feeding trial for them using your patients and pets. While feeding trials, especially on therapeutic diets, cannot be expected to detect all deficiencies or excesses (which may also be due to malabsorption or maldigestion), they give you an added advantage of having someone else evaluate them before you offer them to your clients. Feeding trials are conducted on healthy dogs and cats, with controls that are the same breed and gender. During the trials, the animals must receive the test food as their only source of nutrition. The same formula must be fed throughout the entire trial. The trials are conducted by measuring the daily food consumption, weekly body weight measurement, and stated laboratory parameters measured at the end of the trial, with a complete physical examination by a veterinarian at the beginning and end of the trial, a number of animals not to exceed 25% that can be removed for non-nutritional reasons or poor food intake, and a necropsy conducted on any animal that dies during the trial, with findings recorded. Reproducing animals need the additional following information recorded: body weight within 24 hours of delivery; offspring's body weight within 24 hours of birth; litter size at birth, 1 day later, and at end of study; and any stillborn or congenital abnormalities (Case et al., 2000a, 2000b; Gross et al., 2000a, 2000b, 2000c).

At the end of the feeding trial, the results obtained are compared with the results from a control group, with a historical colony average, or with reference values published by the AAFCO (Case et al., 2000a, 2000b; Gross et al., 2000a, 2000b, 2000c).

All premium manufacturers conduct feeding trials on their foods and continue to conduct them as the foods are changed and updated both for palatability and as new evidence is discovered regarding nutritional requirements. To verify if feeding trails have been conducted on a food, check the product label to find the source of AAFCO certification—if feeding trials have been done, it will be stated on the label as such.

Myth: Pet Food Preservatives Are Bad

"Preservatives" are defined as any substance that is capable of inhibiting or retarding the growth of microorganisms or of masking the evidence of such deterioration (Case et al., 2000c; Gross et al., 2000a, 2000b, 2000c). The primary nutrient requiring protection from preservatives during storage is dietary fat. These fats can be in the form of vegetable oils, animal fats, or the fat-soluble vitamins A, D, E, and K. These nutrients have the potential to undergo oxidative destruction, called lipid peroxidation, during storage. Antioxidants are included in foods to prevent this lipid peroxidation (Case et al., 2000c; Gross et al., 2000a, 2000b, 2000c). Oxidation of fats in pet foods also results in loss of calorie content and the formation of toxic forms of peroxides that can be harmful to the health of pets. The U.S. Food and Drug Administration (FDA) defines an "antioxidant" as any substance that aids in the preservation of foods by retarding deterioration, rancidity, or discoloration as the result of oxidation processes (Case et al., 2000c; Gross et al., 2000a, 2000b, 2000c). Various types of antioxidants have been accepted for use in human and animal foods since 1947. Antioxidants do not reverse the oxidative effects on foods once they have started but rather retard the oxidative process and prevent destruction of the fats in the food. Because of this, antioxidants to be fully effective must be included in the food when it is initially mixed and processed. This inclusion helps prevent rancidity, maintaining the food's flavor, odor, and texture, and prevents accumulation of the toxic end-products of lipid degradation (Case et al., 2000c; Gross et al., 2000a, 2000b, 2000c).

Antioxidants can be divided into two basic types—natural-derived products and synthetic products. Natural-derived products are commonly found in certain grains, vegetable oils, and some herbs and spices. While these products do exist in nature, all of these compounds are processed in some way to make them available for use in commercial foods. The most common natural-derived antioxidants include mixed tocophrols (vitamin E compounds), ascorbic acid (vitamin C), rosemary extract, and citric acid (Case et al., 2000c; Gross et al., 2000a, 2000b, 2000c).

Alpha-tocopherol has the strongest biologic function on tissues but is a poor antioxidant in foods. Delta- and gamma-tocopherols both have low biologic activity but are more effective than alpha-tocopherol as antioxidants. Tocopherols used in foods are obtained primarily from distillation of soybean oil residue. Tocopherols are rapidly decomposed as they protect the fat from oxidation; for this reason, food preserved with mixed tocopherols has a shorter shelf-life than food preserved with a mixture of antioxidants (Case et al., 2000c).

Ascorbic acid (vitamin C) is a water-soluble antioxidant and is not easily soluble with the fatty portion of foods. It does work synergistically with other antioxidants, such as vitamin E and butylated hydroxytoluene. Ascorbyl palminate is similar in structure to ascorbic acid, although it is not normally found in nature. When hydrolyzed, it yields ascorbic acid and the free fatty acid (FFA) palmitic acid, both of which are natural compounds (Case et al., 2000c).

Rosemary extract is obtained from the dried leaves of the evergreen shrub *Rosemarinus officinalis*. It is effective as a natural-derived preservative in high-fat diets and has been shown to enhance antioxidant efficiency when combined with mixed tocopherols, ascorbic acid, and citric acid. Much processing of the plant oil is needed before addition to foods due to the taste associated with the oil, affecting the taste of the food (Case et al., 2000c).

Citric acid is found in citrus fruits such as oranges and lemons and is often included in combination with other natural-derived antioxidants (Case et al., 2000c).

Due to the high cost of using these compounds, they are usually used in conjunction with synthetic antioxidants as preservatives in pet foods. It is difficult to attain the necessary level of natural-derived antioxidants without becoming cost prohibitive (Case et al., 2000c).

Synthetic antioxidants are more effective than natural-derived antioxidants and better withstand the heat, pressure, and moisture during food processing; this is called "carry-through." By being more effective, they better preserve the fat-soluble vitamins A, D, and E for activity in the body rather than in the food (Case et al., 2000c; Gross et al., 2000a, 2000b, 2000c).

Synthetic antioxidants include butylated hydroxyanisole (BHA), butylated hydroxytoluene (BHT), tertiary butylhydroquine (TBHQ), and ethoxyquin. BHA and BHT are approved for use in both human and animal foods and have a synergistic antioxidant effect when used together. BHA and BHT also have good carry-through and a high efficiency in protection of animal fats but are slightly less effective when used with vegetable oils. TBHQ is an effective antioxidant for most fats and is approved for use in human and animal foods in the United States but is not approved for use in Canada, Japan, or the European Economic Community, so it is not usually used in pet foods in the international market. Ethoxyquin has been approved for use in animal feeds for more than 30 years and has been used in pet food manufacturing for more than 15 years. It is approved for both human and animal foods, has good carry-through, and has especially high efficacy in the protection of fats in foods. Ethoxyquin is more efficient as an antioxidant than BHA or BHT, which allows lower levels to be used. It is especially effective in protection of oils that contain high levels of polyunsaturated fatty acids (PUFAs) (Case et al., 2000c; Gross et al., 2000a, 2000b, 2000c).

If the use of synthetic antioxidants is a concern to clients, they should be made aware that most canned foods do not contain antioxidants and that many commercially prepared dry foods use natural-derived antioxidants. There are no studies that support the contention that synthetic antioxidants in general, or ethoxyquin in particular, are responsible for the variety of health problems reported by owners to the FDA. The proper use of antioxidants prevents the occurrence of rancidity and the production of toxic peroxide compounds in foods. In most cases, synthetic antioxidants are the best choice because of their efficacy, good carry-through, and cost. In contrast, poor carry-through, instability, and high levels needed for effective protection make natural-derived antioxidants difficult to use as the sole source in pet foods (Case et al., 2000c; Gross et al., 2000a, 2000b, 2000c).

Conclusion

Once clients are given the facts regarding pet foods, all of our jobs should become easier! After all, a well-informed client is our best friend. With proper information, they will be able to pick a pet food that contains quality ingredients, has undergone feeding trials, and is properly preserved so that all the ingredients are available to their pet. They may also learn that their veterinary team is the best source for nutrition information!

References

Case, L.P., Carey, D.P., Hirakawa, D.A., & Daristotle, L. 2000a. Digestion and absorption. In *Canine and feline nutrition: A resource for companion animal professionals* (2nd. ed., pp. 60–63). St. Louis, MO: Mosby.

Case, L.P., Carey, D.P., Hirakawa, D.A., & Daristotle, L. 2000b. Nutrient content of pet foods. In *Canine and feline nutrition: A resource for companion animal professionals* (2nd. ed., pp. 175–185). St. Louis, MO: Mosby.

Case, L.P., Carey, D.P., Hirakawa, D.A., & Daristotle, L. 2000c. Nutrient content of pet foods. In *Canine and feline nutrition: A resource for companion animal professionals* (2nd. ed., pp. 175–185). St. Louis, MO: Mosby.

Gross, K.L., Wedekind, K.L., Cowell, C.S., Schoenherr,, W.D., Jewell, D.E., Zicker, S.C., Debraekeleer, J., & Frey, R.A. 2000a. Nutrients. In M.S. Hand, C.D. Thatcher, R.L. Remillard, & P. Roudebush (eds.), *Small animal clinical nutrition* (4th. ed., pp. 58–60). Marceline, MO: Walsworth Publishing for Mark Morris Institute.

Gross, K.L., Wedekind, K.L., Cowell, C.S., Schoenherr, W.D., Jewell, D.E., Zicker, S.C., Debraekeleer, J., & Frey, R.A. 2000b. Making commercial pet foods. In M.S. Hand, C.D. Thatcher, R.L. Remillard, & P. Roudebush (eds.), *Small animal clinical nutrition* (4th. ed., pp. 140–146). Marceline, MO: Walsworth Publishing for Mark Morris Institute.

Gross, K.L., Wedekind, K.L., Cowell, C.S., Schoenherr,, W.D., Jewell, D.E., Zicker, S.C., Debraekeleer, J., & Frey, R.A. 2000c. Making pet foods at home. In M.S. Hand, C.D. Thatcher, R.L. Remillard, & P. Roudebush (eds.), *Small animal clinical nutrition* (4th. ed., pp. 167–169). Marceline, MO: Walsworth Publishing for Mark Morris Institute.

30

Nutritional Support

Many hospitalized and critically ill dogs and cats are at risk of becoming severely malnourished because they lack an appetite or the ability to eat. Decreased food intake can be caused by any number of factors ranging from primary medical problems such as diabetes mellitus, inflammatory bowel disease, or chronic renal failure to fear, anxiety, and untreated pain (Buffington et al., 2004).

Who Is at Risk?

Dogs and cats of any age or life stage may become malnourished from inadequate nutrient intake (Remillard et al., 2000). Malnutrition is any disorder with inadequate or unbalanced nutrition that is associated with either nutritional deficiencies or excessive nutrient intakes (Remillard et al., 2000). Protein and energy malnutrition can also result from diets that are inappropriate for the physiologic status of the patient (e.g., low-protein diet when increased protein is required, such as during gestation or lactation) (Remillard et al., 2000).

Insufficient nutrient intake can cause impaired immunity; decreased resistance to infection; inability to withstand shock, surgery, and the effects of drugs; decreased wound strength; muscular weakness; organ failure; and death (Buffington et al., 2004).

Nutrition Goals

The goals of nutritional support are to meet the patients nutritional needs and, if possible, to prevent further deterioration. This can be done by providing protein, carbohydrate, fat, and other nutrients in a formula that can be utilized by the body with maximum efficiency, minimal adverse effects, and minimum discomfort (Donaghue, 1989). When the body uses exogenous (those provided outside of the body) rather than endogenous (those provided by the animal's own body stores) nutrients, the breakdown of lean body mass is slowed down and the patient's response to therapy is optimized (Abood, 1998). Increased protein breakdown in response to illness or injury depletes the body of protein stores, thereby affecting wound healing, immune and cellular functions, and cardiac and respiratory functions (Wingfield, 1997).

When subjected to starvation, body tissue (except the brain and bone) loses cell mass in varying degrees (Donaghue, 1989). Tumors and wounds may act as additional burdens and can further increase the patient's caloric and nutritional requirements (Donaghue, 1989). Malnutrition from inappropriate diets can impair immune function and wound healing, decrease organ function, and affect the prognosis for recovery.

The magnitude of metabolic aberration is determined by the severity of the illness or injury and associated tissue damage (Wingfield, 1997). Even with initiation of adequate nutritional support, muscle wasting and negative nitrogen balance can occur (Wingfield, 1997).

Guidelines for Support

General guidelines for initiating nutritional support include the loss or anticipated loss of more than 10% of the body weight, anorexia for longer than 3 days, trauma, surgery (including elective surgeries), severe systemic infiltrative disease, and increased nutrient loss through diarrhea, vomiting, draining wounds, or burns associated with decreased serum albumin (Wingfield, 1997). Other issues that must be considered include gastrointestinal tract function, whether the patient can tolerate tube or catheter feeding (e.g., presence of any organ failure) and the physical or chemical restraint required for placing the tube or catheter, venous accessibility, whether the patient is at risk for pulmonary aspiration (e.g., megaesophagus), availability of nursing care and equipment, and client cost.

Nutritional Assessment

The cornerstone of nutritional assessment consists of conducting a complete physical examination, obtaining a detailed patient history, recording body weight, assessing the patient's body condition, and evaluating blood chemistry profiles (Abood, 1998). The blood profiles required depend on the patient's condition.

The body condition scores used for healthy animals often do not apply to sick animals. When an animal is physiologically stressed, lean body mass is its preferred energy source; in contrast, healthy animals use stored body fat for energy. The result is increased catabolism of body protein (Buffington et al., 2004).

A patient may present with increased amounts of body fat but be at serious risk of malnutrition-associated complications caused by protein catabolism. Careful examination, including palpation of skeletal muscles over bony prominences (e.g., the scapula, vertebrae, hips, and cranial crest), can help identify any muscle wasting consistent with increase protein catabolism (Remillard et al., 2000). Other indicators of poor nutritional status include edema and ascites, which may reflect low serum protein levels secondary to malnutrition. Poor hair coat and skin condition can also result from inadequate food intake or micronutrient deficiencies (Remillard et al., 2000).

TABLE 30.1. **Nutritional questions.**

- When was the last time your pet ate or drank? How much was offered? How much was consumed?
- What type of food is usually fed (canned, dry, table food, scraps)? How much and how often?
- What brand of food is usually fed? For how long?
- Have there been any recent changes in your pets eating or drinking habits? If so, what changes over what period of time?
- Have there been any recent changes in body condition (e.g., muscle loss, swollen abdomen, hair loss, or poor grooming)?
- Has your pet recently taken, or is currently taking, any medication? Were there any changes in your pet's condition while taking these medications? Is so, what?

From Abood, S.K. 1998. Nutritional assessment of the critical care patient. In *1997 Purina nutrition forum*. St. Louis, MO: Ralston Purina Co.

Calculating Energy Requirements

Caloric requirements are determined by body weight and functions and can be calculated by using the resting energy requirements (RER) for healthy adults at rest in environmentally comfortable cages (Donaghue, 1989). The application of illness factors to the RER are now thought to be a source of more complications rather than improving clinical outcome and are therefore discouraged (Chan, 2005). Water requirements equal those for energy (1 ml = 1 kcal) (Torrance, 1996). Patients that eat more than the calculated RER amounts should not be discouraged from doing so while recovering from surgery or trauma.

Routes of Administration

The gut is generally the safest and most natural route for administering nutrients. Maintaining the intestinal mucosa may also help prevent bacterial translocation from the gut to the rest of the body. This is best accomplished with enteral feeding (Hill, 1994). Voluntary oral intake is the preferred route for enteral nutrition; however, patients must be able to consume at least 85% of their calculated RER for this method of feeding to be effective (Donaghue, 1989; Torrance, 1996). Technicians often need to devise ways to encourage patients to accept oral feedings.

If a patient is unwilling or unable to eat voluntarily, tube feeding should be considered. Tube feeding, however, is limited by diet selections. In most instances, only liquid or gruel diets can be fed through the tube due to the small internal diameter. In addition, tubes can become

TABLE 30.2. **Hints for increasing oral intake of food.**

- Hand-feed or pet the patient during feeding.
- Warm the food to slightly below body temperature, if microwaving be sure food is stirred well before feeding.
- Add warm water to dry food or make a slurry from canned foods by adding warm water.
- Use baby food meats as a top dressing; dogs may also like cat food used as a top dressing.
- Try various shapes and types of bowls. Shallow dishes for cats and brachycephalic dog breeds, plastic may have a strange smell to the animals.
- Use foods that have a strong smell or odor.
- Add appetite stimulants to "jump start" the feeding process (usually ineffective over the long term).

From Torrance, A.G. 1996. Intensive care nutritional support. In N.C. Kelly & J.M. Wills (eds.), *Manual of companion animal nutrition and feeding* (pp. 171–180). Ames, IA: Iowa State Press.

clogged and must be flushed with water frequently to help prevent this (Remillard et al., 2000).

Parenteral Nutrition

When enteral nutrition is not an option as with gut failure, when enteral nutrition could exacerbate a disease (e.g., necrotic hemorrhagic pancreatitis), or the animal's airway cannot be protected and aspiration pneumonia is a concern, parenteral nutrition is an option (Remillard et al., 2000).

Parenteral nutrition uses a modified solution with nutrients that can be absorbed by the cells without passing through the gut first. Parenteral solutions can be used alone or as a supplement to enteral feedings when insufficient caloric intake is seen. Using parenteral nutrition as the only means of calories (total parenteral nutrition [TPN]) is recommended only for patients that cannot be fed enterally; due to expenses and difficulty in obtaining the solutions, short-term use is usually not justified, and most animals will need support for longer than 5 days (Remillard et al., 2000).

Parenteral nutrition has several disadvantages. A dedicated central venous catheter is required, and the special nutrient solution must be properly prepared. Intensive monitoring is necessary, and thrombophlebitis and sepsis are serious complications if strict aseptic technique is not followed (Tennant, 1996). Lack of nutrients in the intestinal lumen may lead to breakdown of the bacterial barrier in the gut, further increasing the incidence of sepsis (Donaghue, 1989). A transitional period is necessary to wean the patient from parenteral to enteral feedings (Donaghue, 1989).

Because parenteral solutions have very high osmolality (often greater than 800 to 1,200 mOsm), a central venous catheter should be used to prevent phlebitis. If a peripheral catheter is used, the solutions must be substantially diluted to decrease the osmolality, also diluting the caloric content. Administration must also be adjusted to prevent fluid overload (Tennant, 1996). Line separation or breakage must be avoided to decrease the incidence of introducing bacteria to the solution (Tennant, 1996).

Diets

Patients with stress starvation can be glucose intolerant and, if so, use glucose less efficiently as an energy source. Therefore, protein and fat are important sources of energy (Tennant, 1996). Before evaluating the need for fat, protein, and carbohydrate, however, a good diet strategy should address the animal's requirement for water and correct any

TABLE 30.3. **Practices that adversely affect nutritional status.**

- Failing to record weight daily
- Failing to observe, measure, and record amounts of food consumed
- Allowing diffusion of responsibility for patient care during staff rotation
- Prolonging administration of dextrose- and electrolyte-containing solution without providing additional nutritional support
- Delaying nutritional support until a patient reaches an advanced state
- Withholding food to conduct multiple diagnostic tests or procedures
- Failing to recognize and treat increased nutritional needs
- Failing to appreciate the role of nutrition in prevention and recovery from infection and placing unwarranted reliance on drugs
- Allowing surgery to be performed without verifying whether the patient is optimally nourished
- Providing inadequate nutritional support after surgery
- Failing to use laboratory tests to assess nutritional status

From Remillard, R., Armstrong, P.J., & Davenport, D. 2000. Assisted feeding in hospitalized patients: Enteral and parenteral nutrition. In M.S. Hand, C.D. Thatcher, R.L. Remillard, & P. Roudebush (eds.), *Small animal clinical nutrition* (4th. ed., pp. 352–370). Marceline, MO: Walsworth Publishing for Mark Morris Institute.

preexisting fluid and acid-base deficits (Tennant, 1996). After these needs have been satisfied, sufficient fat, carbohydrate, and protein should be provided to meet the animal's energy requirements and minimize the gluconeogenesis of amino acids (Tennant, 1996).

Commercial pet foods are specifically designed to meet the dietary requirements of cats and dogs and contain ingredients (e.g., glutamine, taurine, carnitine) not usually found in liquid or parenteral diets (Tennant, 1996). The principal differences between human and animal liquid diets are the extent that ingredients are subject to hydrolysis and the protein contents (Tennant, 1996). For example, most human enteral diets contain 14% to 17% protein, which is insufficient for both dogs and cats. In addition, arginine and methionine levels in human enteral diets tend to be too low, especially for cats (Tennant, 1996).

Pediatric or growth pet diets are often recommended because they are highly digestible, have high fat and protein contents, and are very

TABLE 30.4. **Recommended levels of protein, fat, and carbohydrate in critical care diets.**

Species	Protein (% ME)	Fat (% ME)	Carbohydrate (% ME)
Dogs	20–30	30–55	15–50
Cats	25–35	40–55	15–25

From Tennant, B. 1996. Feeding the sick animal. In N.C. Kelly & J.M. Wills (eds.), *Manual of companion animal nutrition and feeding* (pp. 181–186). Ames, IA: Iowa State Press.

palatable (Hill, 1994). Meat-based baby foods contain 30% to 70% protein and 20% to 60% fat. However, because they are deficient in calcium, vitamin A, and thiamine, baby foods should not be used as the sole dietary source (Wingfield, 1997).

Rate of Diet Initiation

Because nutritional support is not an emergency procedure, the general guidelines are to start slowly (Hill, 1994). Food intake should be gradually increased over a 2 to 3 day period until the estimated caloric intake is met (Tennant, 1996). If the patient shows discomfort, vomits, is nauseous, or becomes distressed, the diet and the route and rate of delivery need to be assessed.

Generally, 50% of the RER, divided into multiple small meals, is offered the first day. If this amount is well tolerated, then 100% of the RER can be fed the second day. If the feedings are not well tolerated, the increases should be more gradual over the next 2 to 3 days. Smaller meals tend to be better tolerated because they do not cause overdistention of the stomach and subsequent delayed gastric emptying or aggravate nausea, as can occur with larger meals (Remillard et al., 2000). Sometimes with patients receiving assisted feedings via nasoesophageal, esophageal, or gastrostomy tube, delivering the food using a syringe pump for a continuous-rate infusion will allow more food to be fed than if bolus feedings were used. It also will significantly decrease the incidence of nausea, because only small amounts of food are in the stomach at any given time. This also is much easier on the nursing staff than if frequent small bolus feedings are being fed every 2 to 4 hours.

The refeeding syndrome, an electrolyte disturbance that can occur in patients with depleted intracellular ions (e.g. potassium, phosphorus, magnesium, and calcium), can be seen with malnutrition, starvation as with feline hepatic lipidosis, or prolonged diuresis as seen with uncontrolled diabetes or renal failure. Patients at greatest risk are those severely malnourished with significant loss of lean body mass. Reintroduction of nutrition results in a rapid shift of these ions from the serum (where levels may be normal before feeding) to the intracellular space. Profound hypophosphatemia, hypokalemia, and/or hypomagnesemia may result and can lead to muscle weakness, intravascular hemolysis, and possibly cardiac and respiratory failure. The syndrome can be avoided by monitoring the patient closely, introducing feeding cautiously (continuous-rate infusion of a commercial recovery diet), monitoring electrolytes frequently (every 12 to 24 hours), and supplementing the diet as needed (Donaghue, 1989).

Implementing Feeding Orders

Technicians responsible for patient treatments should be given instructions listing the type of food to be offered along with how much to give
and how often. A flowchart can be used to record the amount eaten, the
technique used to feed the patient, and the food that was offered (e.g.,
"$\frac{1}{2}$ can of slightly warmed dog food offered by hand at 3:00 p.m., ate
well"). The technician can then draw a circle on the flowchart and fill in
the amount of food the patient consumed (e.g., filling in one quarter of
the circle if the patient ate $\frac{1}{4}$ of the amount offered); if the patient
refused to eat, the technician should record an "R" in the circle. The
technician should also note whether any food, amount, or technique
recorded differs from the instructions. Such record-keeping provides veterinarians with an accurate measurement of food intake and technicians
with feeding methods that succeed on a per-patient basis, which is especially helpful during shift changes.

Diet Transitions

Although diet transitions may occur while the patient is hospitalized,
typically this is done 2 to 6 weeks after discharge from the hospital.
Transition depends on the diet being fed, condition of the patient, its
response to therapy, and the comfort level of the owner. As with diet
initiation, it is best to proceed slowly. For example, when shifting from
a support diet to a maintenance diet, each dietary change should represent an additional one quarter of the current diet every 3 to 4 days. For
days 1 to 4, feed $\frac{3}{4}$ of the therapeutic diet and $\frac{1}{4}$ of the maintenance
diet; days 5 to 8, feed $\frac{1}{2}$ of the therapeutic diet and $\frac{1}{2}$ of the maintenance diet; days 9 to 12, feed $\frac{1}{4}$ of the therapeutic diet and $\frac{3}{4}$ of the
maintenance diet; and day 13, feed 100% maintenance diet (i.e., tran-
sition phase of 12 to 16 days). If a problem develops at any stage, the
owners should be instructed to return to the last diet combination that
worked.

Technicians should supply owners with well-written, concise discharge instructions and reasonable expectation of what the diet being
fed can do. Unfortunately, therapeutic diets cannot "cure" inflammatory
bowel disease, chronic renal failure, or diabetes, although they are often
used to help control the signs of these diseases. It is very important that
owners are aware of this.

TABLE 30.5. Sample flowchart showing accurate food intake notes.

Conclusion

Being aware of the nutritional aspects of patient care can improve the long-term outcome of the patient's health as well as the client–patient–veterinary team relationship. Technicians can assume a primary role in providing excellent nutritional support to our patients. Even if we are not able to save our patients every time, the clients understand that we do care and want what is best for their pet.

References

Abood, S.K. 1998. Nutritional assessment of the critical care patient. In *1997 Purina nutrition forum*. St. Louis, MO: Ralston Purina Co.

Buffington, T., Holloway, C.A., & Abood, S.K. 2004. Nornal dogs. In *Manual of veterinary dietetics* (pp. 54–60). St. Louis, MO: Elsevier.

Chan, D.L. 2005. In-hospital starvation: Inadequate nutritional support. In *11th International Veterinary Emergency & Critical Care Symposium proceedings* (pp. 515–518). Produced through sponsorship of Hill's and Pfizer.

Donaghue, S. 1989. Nutritional support of hospitalized patients. *The Veterinary Clinics of North America. Small Animal Practice, 19*, 475–493.

Hill, Richard C. 1994. Critical care nutrition. In J.M. Wills & K.W. Simpson (eds.), *The Waltham book of clinical nutrition of the dog and cat* (pp. 39–57). Tarrytown, NY: Pergamon Press.

Remillard, R., Armstrong, P.J., & Davenport, D. 2000. Assisted feeding in hospitalized patients: Enteral and parenteral nutrition. In M.S. Hand, C.D. Thatcher, R.L. Remillard, & P. Roudebush (eds.), *Small animal clinical nutrition* (4th. ed., pp. 352–370). Marceline, MO: Walsworth Publishing for Mark Morris Institute.

Tennant, B. 1996. Feeding the sick animal. In N.C. Kelly & J.M. Wills (eds.), *Manual of companion animal nutrition and feeding* (pp. 181–186). Ames, IA: Iowa State Press.

Torrance, A.G. 1996. Intensive care nutritional support. In N.C. Kelly & J.M. Wills (eds.), *Manual of companion animal nutrition and feeding* (pp. 171–180). Ames, IA: Iowa State Press.

Wingfield, W.E. 1997. The essentials of life in critically ill animals. In *Purina nutrition forum*. St. Louis, MO: Ralston Purina Co.

31

Assisted Feeding in Dogs and Cats

Addressing the nutritional needs of our hospitalized and critical care patients can dramatically improve their outcomes, but also allows them to return home sooner. Oral enteral nutrition is the ideal route, but if the patient is unable or unwilling to consume at least 85% of their calculated resting energy requirements (RER), then another route needs to be used.

When oral nutrition is not an option, what are the other options? There are a number of feeding tube options available. The choice of tube will be dependent on the condition of the patient, the disease being addressed, expense of administration, availability of intensive care facilities, preferred food, and anticipated length of feeding assistance.

The first step is to calculate the RER for the individual patient. The most widely used formula is: (weight in kilograms $\times$ 30) + 70 = RER.

This formula can be used in both cats and dogs over 2 kg to 45 kg (Hand et al., 2000; Marks, 2000; Willard, 1992). For animals outside this range, one of the logarithmic formulas can be used to calculate RER.

The best feeding tubes for prolonged use are made of polyurethane or silicone. For short-term feeding, usually less than 10 days, polyvinylchloride (PVC) tubes can be used. These are not appropriate for long-term feeding because they tend to become stiff with prolonged use, causing additional discomfort for the patient. Silicone is softer and more flexible than other tube materials and has a greater tendency to stretch and collapse. Polyurethane is stronger than silicone, allowing for thinner tube walls and a greater internal diameter, despite the same

TABLE 31.1. Tube feeding comparisons.

Type of tube	Condition	Disease	Intensive care unit costs	Food type used	Length of time
Nasoesophageal/ nasogastric	Not recommended for patients that are vomiting or have respiratory disease	Short-term anorexia, supplement oral intake	$	Liquid ± thinning required; CRI or bolus	Short-term, in-hospital use only (3–7 days)
Pharyngostomy/ esophagostomy	Not recommended for patients that are vomiting or have respiratory disease	Hepatic lipidosis, anorexia, oral surgery or trauma, cancer	SS	Liquid, recovery diet or gruel commercial diet based on tube size; CRI or bolus	Long-term, in-hospital and at-home use (1–20 weeks, depending on tube type used)
Gastrostomy	Can be used on patients that are vomiting or that have respiratory disease	Pancreatitis, hepatic lipidosis, anorexia, esophageal strictures, oral surgery or trauma, cancer	SSS	Liquid, recovery diet or gruel commercial diet based on tube size; CRI or bolus	Long-term use, can be permanent, depending on tube type used
Jejunostomy	Can be used on patients that are vomiting or that have respiratory disease	Pancreatitis, intestinal anastomosis, coma	$$$$	Liquid diet; CRI or bolus	Short-term, in-hospital use only (3–10 days)

222

French size. Both the silicone and polyurethane tubes do not disintegrate or become brittle in situ, providing a longer tube life. The French unit measures the outer lumen diameter of a tube and is equal to 0.33 mm (Marks, 2000).

While force feeding can be used to provide the necessary nutrition, this is usually too stressful to the patient, not to mention the stress to the owner. Seldom is this method able to deliver the volume of nutrients necessary to meet the patient's needs.

Nasoesophageal/Nasogastric Tube Placement

Nasoesophageal tubes are useful for providing short-term nutritional support, usually less than 10 days. They can be used in patients with a functional esophagus, stomach, and intestines. Nasoesophageal tubes are contraindicated in patients that are vomiting or comatose or lack a gag reflex (Guilford et al., 1996; Marks, 2000).

Supplies needed include lidocaine drops (ophthalmic drops can be used); 5 to 8 Fr tube with length sufficient to reach the distal esophagus, sterile lubricant, suture or glue, Luer slip catheter plug, and Elizabethan collar.

The length of tube to be inserted is determined by measuring from the nasal planum along the side of the patient to the caudal margin of the last rib. This indicates the ideal tube placement—mark this area with either a piece of tape or other marker. After instilling a few drops of the lidocaine into the nose, a sterile catheter of sufficient length (8 Fr × 42 inch in dogs >15 kg, 5 Fr × 36 inch in dogs <15 kg) is advanced into the nose. The tube should be passed with the tip directed in a caudoventral, medial direction into the ventrolateral aspect of the external nares. The head should be held in a normal static position. As soon as the tip of the catheter reaches the medial septum at the floor of the nasal cavity in dogs, the external nares are pushed dorsally; this opens the ventral meatus, ensuring passage of the tube into the oropharynx. In cats, the tube can be inserted initially in a ventromedial direction and continued directly into the oropharynx. The tube is inserted until the tape tab or marked area is reached. To evaluate proper tube placement, 3 to 15ml of sterile water or saline can be injected through the tube and the animal evaluated for coughing. Coughing would indicate the tube is placed in the lungs, not in the esophagus. Lateral radiographs may also be taken to confirm tube location. After confirmation of position, the tube is secured with either glue or sutures at the external nares and along the dorsal midline along the bridge of the nose. Continue to direct the tube over the head and secure with a bandage around the neck. Place the catheter plug into the catheter. An Elizabethan collar is used in most animals to prevent inadvertent removal of the tube (Guilford et al., 1996; Hand et al., 2000; Marks, 2000; Willard, 1992).

Complications include epistaxis, lack of tolerance of the procedure, and inadvertent removal by the patient. These tubes should not be used in vomiting patients or those with respiratory disease (Guilford et al., 1996; Hand et al., 2000; Marks, 2000; Willard, 1992).

To place a nasogastric tube, follow the same procedure but measure the length to 3 to 4 inches past the last rib. Nasogastric tubes increase the risk of gastroesophageal reflux, increasing the incidence of esophageal strictures.

Due to the small internal diameter of these tubes, only liquid enteral diets can be used. They can be either fed through a syringe pump as a continuous-rate infusion or bolus fed. If feeding through a syringe pump, completely change the delivery equipment every 24 hours to help prevent bacterial growth within the system. Tube clogging is a common problem; a syringe pump may help to decrease the incidence, as will flushing well before and after bolus feeding. If the tube becomes clogged, replacement may be necessary. Diluting the liquid with water may also help, although this further decreases the caloric concentration of the diet, increasing the volume necessary to meet the caloric needs.

When removing, the tube may be simply pulled out after the glue or sutures are removed.

Pharyngostomy Tube Placement

With the increased use of gastrostomy tubes, the indications for the use of pharyngostomy tubes are few and far between (Guilford et al., 1996; Hand et al., 2000; Marks, 2000; Willard, 1992). The indications for pharyngostomy tubes are similar to those for nasoesophageal tubes, except pharyngostomy tube placement requires anesthesia.

Supplies needed include an appropriately sized tube, forceps, scalpel blade, suture or tape to secure, and Luer slip catheter plug.

The patient is anesthetized, intubated, and positioned in lateral recumbency. The area caudal to the mandible is clipped and surgically prepped. A 14 to 18 Fr PVC tube is premeasured as with a nasoesophageal tube and marked, except that the tube entrance should be caudal to the mandible. The mouth is held open with a speculum, and the hyoid apparatus is palpated with one finger. The tube exit site must be carefully planned to avoid interfering with the laryngeal opening and epiglottic movement. The tube should exit as far caudally and dorsally along the lateral pharyngeal wall as possible. The finger in the mouth locates the hyoid apparatus and protrudes from the pharyngeal wall laterally at the exit site. Forceps can also be used to locate the tube exit site. A 1 cm skin incision is made over the bulging pharyngeal wall; long, curved forceps are used to bluntly tunnel caudally through the tissue from outside to inside. Blunt dissection prevents injury to nearby nerves, carotid artery, and jugular vein. Forceps are used to grasp one end of the feeding tube so it exits through the dissection site while the other end is passed down the esophagus. The tube is then secured to the skin with tape and sutures. Place the catheter plug into the catheter (Hand et al., 2000).

Complications include airway obstruction, tube displacement damage to the cervical nerves and blood vessels, and infection at the exit site. Improper placement caudal to the hyoid apparatus can result in airway obstruction or aspiration. These tubes should not be used in vomiting patients or those with respiratory disease (Guilford et al., 1996; Hand et al., 2000; Marks, 2000; Willard, 1992).

Because these tubes tend to have a larger diameter than nasoesophageal tubes, a gruel recovery diet can be used if the tube size is greater than 8 Fr. These diets may still need to be thinned with water to aid in passage through the tube.

When removing the tube, it may be simply pulled out after the sutures are removed. The exit hole is allowed to heal by second intention. A light bandage may be applied for the first 12 hours.

Esophagostomy Tube Placement

Esophagostomy tube placement does require anesthesia to perform; the patient should be anesthetized, intubated, and placed in lateral recumbency. The entire lateral cervical region from ventral midline to near dorsal midline is clipped and surgically prepped.

Supplies needed include large Kelly or Carmalt forceps, appropriately sized tube, tape or suture to secure, scalpel blade, and Luer slip catheter plug.

One technique uses a large curved Kelly or Carmalt forceps inserted into the proximal cervical esophagus. The tip of the forceps is turned laterally and pressure is applied in an outward direction, causing a bulge in the cervical tissue so the instrument tip can be seen and palpated externally. A small skin incision, just large enough to accommodate the feeding tube, is made over the tip of the forceps. In small dogs and cats, the tip of the forceps is forced bluntly through the esophagus; in larger dogs, a deeper incision is made to allow passage of the tip of the forceps through the esophagus. The tube is premeasured as with a nasoesophageal tube, except the exit is in the mid to caudal esophagus. The distal tip of the tube is grasped with the forceps, pulled in to the esophagus and out through the mouth, and then turned around and redirected into the esophagus. The tube is secured with tape and sutures. A light bandage is applied around the neck with triple antibiotic ointment applied at the tube site. Place the catheter plug into the catheter (Guilford et al., 1996; Hand et al., 2000; Marks, 2000; Willard, 1992).

There are also tube placement systems available for esophagostomy tube placement.

Complications include tube displacement due to vomiting or removal by the patient, skin infection around the exit site, and biting off of the tube end by the patient after vomiting.

Depending on the technique used and the size of the patient, an 8 to 20 Fr catheter may be used; the large bore of these catheters allows for feeding of a gruel recovery diet, sometimes without dilution with water. These catheters are also easy for clients to use and maintain as long as vomiting is not a problem.

When removing the tube, it may be simply pulled out after the sutures are removed. The exit hole is allowed to heal by second intention. A light bandage may be applied for the first 12 hours.

Gastrostomy Tube Placement

Gastrostomy tubes can be placed either endoscopically, blindly, or surgically. All three techniques require general anesthesia. Endoscopic placement allows for visualization of the esophagus and stomach, as well as biopsy collection from the stomach and proximal duodenum and foreign body removal. Blind biopsy allows placement of a gastrostomy tube without the investment in an endoscopic unit. Surgical placement is useful during surgical exploratory or when the scope cannot be passed through the esophagus due to trauma or esophageal strictures.

Supplies needed include an endoscope, endoscopic grabbers, Pezzer catheter, 14-gauge needle or catheter, one or two lengths of No. 2 suture material about 3 feet long, catheter guide, sterile lubricant, scalpel blade, and Luer slip catheter plug.

For percutaneous endoscopic gastrostomy (PEG) tube placement, the patient is anesthetized and placed in right lateral recumbency. The right flank is clipped and surgically prepped from 1 to 2 inches above the last caudal rib to 2 to 3 inches beyond the last caudal rib. The area should be 4 to 6 inches in diameter. A 20 to 24 Fr Pezzer catheter is used for placement; these are available singly and as kits. The endoscope in advanced into the stomach and used to insufflate air into it. This helps to ensure that the spleen or omentum does not become entrapped between the stomach and body wall. An assistant digitally palpates the external body wall about 1 to 2 cm behind the ninth rib; the palpation can be seen internally and can be used to confirm correct placement of the feeding tube. When the site is confirmed, a 14-gauge needle or catheter is introduced into the stomach through the body wall, a length of No. 2 suture is threaded through the needle into the stomach and grasped with endoscopic grabbers, and the string and scope are removed from the stomach. Ensure that the assistant maintains a hold on his or her end of the suture and that it does not become pulled thorough as the scope is removed. The catheter guide is slid onto the suture and used to secure the Pezzer catheter (it helps to bevel the end of the Pezzer catheter to help it fit into the catheter guide). Using the 14-gauge needle, push it through the Pezzer catheter and then thread the suture through the needle, remove the needle, and secure the suture. Pull everything taut, apply the sterile lubricant to the feeding tube liberally, and, using firm and steady pressure, pull the catheter guide with Pezzer catheter attached through the body wall—it may be necessary to use a scalpel blade to enlarge the hole in the body wall to allow passage of the tube assembly. It is important to maintain firm and steady pressure throughout the entire passage of the feeding tube from the mouth through the body wall. Once the tube is through the body wall, pull the mushroom tip firmly against the stomach wall; in most animals, this can be felt from the outside. An external tube assemble should be made to prevent the tube from migrating back into the stomach, be sure to leave a little extra room (about 1 inch) to allow tube movement and weight gain. Place the Luer plug into the catheter (Guilford et al., 1996; Hand et al., 2000; Marks, 2000; Willard, 1992).

A minimum of 12 hours is needed for a temporary stoma to form before feeding can begin. The feeding tube should be left in place for a minimum of 7 to 10 days to allow a permanent stoma to form before removal. The tubes can be left in long term (1 to 6 months) without replacement. When replaced with another PEG tube, low-profile silicone tube, or Foley-type feeding tube, the stoma can be used for the rest of the patient's life. Complications associated with PEG tubes include those seen from tube placement such as splenic laceration, gastric hemorrhage, and pneumoperitoneum. Delayed complications can also be seen, such as vomiting, aspiration pneumonia, tube removal, tube migration, and peritonitis and stoma infection (Marks, 2000).

Blind percutaneous gastrostomy tube placement involves basically the same technique as endoscopic placement, but a large plastic or steel tube is used instead of the endoscope and a firm wire is used instead of the suture. The catheter is the same as in the endoscopic insertion technique. Reported complications are the same as for PEG tubes, although the risk of splenic, stomach, or omental laceration is greater. Contraindications to using the blind technique include severe obesity, which would make palpation of the end of the tube difficult and esophageal disease.

Surgical placement has been largely superseded by endoscopic placement because of the ease and speed of placement, lower cost, and decreased morbidity. A surgical approach may be indicated in obese animals, those with esophageal disease, or when laparotomy is already scheduled. To place a surgical gastrostomy, a larger incision is needed into the stomach and the exit location is sometimes hard to locate because of the position on the surgical table. Surgical placement involves placing purse string sutures around the catheter to secure it as well as attaching the stomach to the body wall.

Gastrostomy tube placement is the technique of choice for long-term enteral support. These tubes are well tolerated by the patient, produce minimal discomfort, allow feeding of either gruel recovery diets or blenderized commercial foods, and can be easily managed by owners at home (Guilford et al., 1996). Patients are able to eat normally with gastrostomy tubes in placed and can easily be used as a nutritional supplement until the patient is totally self-feeding. For patients that are difficult to medicate and require long-term medications, many medicines can also be given through the feeding tube. The major disadvantage of gastrostomy tubes is the need for general anesthesia and the risk of peritonitis (Guilford et al., 1996).

For animals requiring long-term management, the initial Pezzer catheter can be replaced with either low-profile silicone tubes or with Foley-type gastrostomy tubes. Both of these types can be placed through the external stoma site without the endoscope. Sedation or anesthesia may be necessary based on the individual patient.

For removal, if the tube has been in place 16 weeks or less, the tube may be simply removed. This is best accomplished by placing the patient in right lateral recumbency. The tube is grasped with the right hand close to the body wall, with the left hand holding the animal. Pull firmly and consistently to the right in an upward motion. Some force may be required for this. It is also helpful to ensure that the patient has been fasted and to place a towel over the tube site to catch any "stuff." If the tube has been in longer than 16 weeks, the incidence of tube breakage is much higher. Depending on where the breakage occurs, the remaining tube pieces may need to be endoscopically retrieved. Larger patients can easily pass retained parts; smaller patients may need to have them retrieved.

The exit hole is allowed to heal by second intention. A light bandage may be applied for the first 12 hours.

Jejunostomy Tube Placement

Jejunostomy feeding is indicated when the upper gastrointestinal tract must be rested or when pancreatic stimulation must be decreased. Jejunal tubes can be placed either surgically or threaded through a gastrostomy tube for transpyloric placement. Standard gastrojejunal tubes designed for humans are unreliable in dogs due to frequent reflux of the jejunal portion of the tube back into the stomach. Investigation is ongoing involving endoscopic placement of transpyloric jejunal tubes through PEG tubes.

Supplies needed for placement include 5 to 8 Fr PVC tubing, suture, and Luer slip catheter plug.

Due to the small diameter of these tubes and the location, liquid enteral diets are recommended. Because the jejunum has minimal storage capacity compared with the stomach, continuous-rate infusion using a syringe pump is the preferred method of delivery.

Common complications include osmotic diarrhea and vomiting. It is recommended that the jejunal tube be left in place for 7 to 10 days to allow adhesions to form around the tube site and prevent leakage back into the abdomen (Guilford et al., 1996; Willard, 1992). Completely changing the delivery equipment every 24 hours will help prevent bacterial growth within the system. Clogging is a common problem; a syringe pump may help to decrease the incidence as will flushing well every 4 hours.

When removing the tube, it may be simply pulled out after the sutures are removed. The exit hole is allowed to heal by second intention. A light bandage may be applied for the first 12 hours.

Conclusion

The enteral route is the preferred method of nutritional support in patients with functional gastrointestinal tracts. Many tube and food choices are available and can be tailored to fit the individual patient and condition. Providing our patients with nutritional support should not be treated as an afterthought.

References

Guilford, W.G., Center, S.A., & Strombeck, D.R. 1996. Nutritional management of gastrointestinal disease. In W.G. Guilford, S.A. Center, D.R. Strombeck, D. Williams, & D. Meyer (eds.), *Strombeck's small animal gastroenterology* (3rd. ed., pp. 904–908). Philadelphia: W.B. Saunders.

Hand, M.S., Thatcher, C.D., Remillard, R.L., & Roudebush, P. 2000. Appendix V: Assisted feeding techniques. In *Small animal clinical nutrition* (4th. ed., pp. 1145–1153). Marceline, MO: Walsworth Publishing for Mark Morris Institute.

Marks, S.L. 2000. Enteral and parenteral nutritional support. In S.J. Ettinger & E.C. Feldman (eds.), *Textbook of veterinary internal medicine, Volume 1* (5th. ed., pp. 275–282). Philadelphia: W.B. Saunders.

Willard, M. 1992. The gastrointestinal system. In R.W. Nelson & C.G. Couto (eds.), *Essentials of small animal internal medicine* (pp. 305–309). St. Louis, MO: Mosby.

Noncompany Sites of interest

American Feed Industry Associates
www.afia.org
Association of American Feed Control Officials
www.aafco.org
Food and Drug Administration
www.fda.gov
Pet Food Institute
www.petfoodinstitute.org
United States Department of Agriculture
www.usda.gov
Pet Food Database
www.balanceit.com

Provides a database of more than 3,000 pet foods, allowing for comparison of various foods, and calculates nutrient distribution and metabolizable energy. Can also be used for formulate homemade diets. Designed and run by a boarded-certified veterinary nutritionist.

Pet Food Companies

Bil-Jac Foods
www.bil-jac.com

Dad's Pet Care
www.dadsproducts.com
Del Monte Corporation
www.delmonte.com
Diamond
www.diamondpet.com
Eagle
www.eaglepack.com
Hill's Pet Nutrition
www.hillspet.com
Iams Company
www.iams.com
Kent Feeds
www.kentfeeds.com
Kraft Foods North America
www.kraft.com
Masterfoods USA
www.waltham.com
Meow Mix Company
www.meowmix.com
Natural Balance Pet Foods
www.naturalbalanceinc.com
Nestle Purina Pet Care
www.purina.com
Nutro Products
www.nutroproducts.com
Old Mother Hubbard
www.omhpet.com
Pro-Pet
www.propet.com
Royal Canin
www.royalcanin.us

This is not an all-inclusive list of pet food companies, and sites as well as companies are subject to change without notice. These companies are members of the Pet Food Institute and have provided website addresses.